365
ENERGY
BOOSTERS

Jayne
Live it up!
Katrina

365
ENERGY
BOOSTERS

Juice Up Your Life,
Thump Your Thymus,
Wiggle as Much as Possible,
Rev Up with Red,
Brush Your Body,
Do a Spinal Rock,
Pop a Pumpkin Seed

CONARI PRESS

First published in 2005 by Conari Press,
an imprint of Red Wheel/Weiser, LLC
York Beach, ME
With offices at:
368 Congress Street
Boston, MA 02210
www.redwheelweiser.com

Library of Congress Cataloging-in-Publication Data
Seton, Susannah
   365 energy boosters : juice up your life, thump your thymus, wiggle as
much as possible, rev up with red, brush your body, do a spinal rock, pop
a pumpkin seed / Susannah Seton and Sondra Kornblatt.
       p. cm.
   Includes bibliographical references.
   ISBN 1-57324-869-X
   1. Health. 2. Vitality. 3. Fatigue—Prevention. 4. Mental
fatigue—Prevention. I. Title: Three hundred sixty-five energy boosters.
II. Kornblatt, Sondra. III. Title.

RA776.5.S435 2005
613—dc22
2005013603

Typeset in Minion, Mrs. Eaves, and Pike by Jill Feron/FeronDesign
Printed in Canada
FR

12 11 10 09 08 07 06 05
 8 7 6 5 4 3 2 1

Energy is all there is! Remember the parable in the Bible about the man who sells all he has to buy the one "pearl of great price"? Your true energy is this pearl.
—Tae Yun Kim

NOTE TO READERS

INTRODUCTION

Tired of Feeling Tired?

Energy is eternal delight.
—William Blake

A friend with four kids under the age of seven and a full-time job recently had to go into the hospital for minor surgery. "I'm actually looking forward to it," he confided. "Finally I can get some rest."

I know the feeling, don't you? Whatever our circumstances, no matter our age, we're all working longer and harder—and feeling the effects. According to HealthFocus International, an organization that tracks health trends, more than half of women between the ages of eighteen and forty-eight complain of lack of energy.

I know that was true for me. I'd been dragging for years when I had the idea to finally do something about it. I'd write a book on the best ways to get more energy! That's how I learn—collecting tips for books and trying them out. There was only one problem—I was so tired that it felt daunting to do it on my own. Having done a "365" book before, I knew how much work it takes.

Then I met Sondra Kornblatt, a writer specializing in sleep and wellness. Immediately I realized that she would be the perfect collaborator—we could divvy up the task. And so we did.

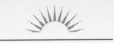

And in the process, I learned many ways to restore and rejuvenate my body, mind, and spirit. Now, after trying many of the boosters in this book, I sleep better and have more energy for what really matters to me. I also learned what my daily energy pattern was—I no longer expect it to remain steady throughout the day and thus don't think there is something "wrong" with me.

But don't take my word for it; try some for yourself. You will find that we offer a huge variety of approaches—some mental, some emotional, others physical. That's because the life force that we call energy is influenced by all those domains, and the reasons we feel low energy can be from any number of physical, emotional, or mental strains.

You'll find suggestions for exercises, for supplements, for getting organized, for meditations, for energy-boosting aromas, and food. You'll discover ideas for getting real rest, for ruling out environmental problems like mold, for one-minute energizing moves at your desk, and hundreds more. All of these are *suggestions*—not meant to substitute for medical advice, for fatigue can be a symptom of serious illness. You can't possibly do them all—that's exhausting even to contemplate—nor are you meant to. There are 365 so that you can pick and choose the approaches that seem right to you. As you read through, notice what ideas jump out at you. Pick one or two of those. Then commit to doing them for a couple weeks and track the effect. If it's working, great. If not, try something else.

Just don't try too many at once because it will be difficult to know which method is actually working for you.

It is my hope that you find ideas in here that will put a spring back into your step and the feeling of zest back into your life. Energy is your most precious human resource. Without it, you simply go through the motions of your life. With it, you have the oomph to passionately engage in your work and your relationships, and experience the simple joy of being alive that is your birthright.

—SUSANNAH SETON

Understand Energy Cycles

Energy ebbs and flows during the day. In his book *Calm Energy*, mood scientist Robert E. Thayer cites research that shows how energy typically follows a pattern: low upon waking, rising to a high in late morning or early afternoon, declining in the afternoon, perhaps with a slight rise in early evening, followed by a steady decline until bedtime.

This information can be liberating. You're not supposed to feel perky all day long—it's natural for it to ebb and flow! Once you understand this, you can stop feeling something is wrong with you when you feel low energy in the late afternoon and evening. It's your biorhythms—and it happens to everyone, with slight variations. Now doesn't that make you feel better?

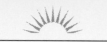

Track Your Energy/Tension Cycles

In *Calm Energy*, Robert Thayer points out that in addition to natural energy cycles we also have tension cycles: tension tends to be lowest when waking, and increases throughout the day, reaching a peak at about five p.m. "The relationship between energy and tension is critical for understanding our everyday behavior," he writes. "When our energy is high, we can withstand stress with relative impunity. But as our energy drops, stress can have its greatest effect.... One negative effect of this period of tense tiredness is that we often do things we would prefer not to do to self-regulate the unpleasant state." Things like eating or drinking, or not exercising.

ENERGY
BOOSTER

2

When you put the two cycles together, in general, between ten a.m. and one p.m. is a time of the highest energy and lowest tension, the perfect time to do challenging tasks. If you are interested in tracking your specific cycles, you need to do it for three days. Pick typical days when you go to bed and get up at regular times and face ordinary tasks. Rate yourself on the hour, every hour from waking to sleeping on a scale of 1 to 10 for energy (1 being lowest) and a separate scale for tension (1 being lowest). Use a kitchen timer to remind yourself to do it.

After three days, look at when your energy is the highest and tension the lowest. This is your peak performance time. Also look at when tension is highest and energy lowest. These are the times you are the most vulnerable to overeating or other unwanted behaviors. Then you can plan to use a more healthy energy booster or take a siesta.

Air Out Your Dry Cleaning

The cleaning fluids used to clean your clothes could be making you tired. Some can cause the thyroid to stop working properly. To avoid giving yourself a chemical blast, air your clean clothes outside. When that chemical smell is gone, it means the solvents have evaporated and it is safe to bring your clothes into the house.

What Your Fatigue Is Trying to Tell You

Debra Waterhouse suggests in *Outsmarting Female Fatigue* that we just write the question out—"What is my fatigue trying to tell me?"—and notice what comes up for an answer. There are no wrong answers, but in doing this, avoid blaming yourself: "It's telling me it's all my fault." Also don't assume that it means you have a dread disease. What you discover will help you decide which other ideas in this book you might want to try.

Make an Energy Elixir

When you hit the mid-afternoon slump, try a smoothie made with tea. It gives you a bit of a caffeine boost but at only half the strength of a cup of coffee, and it won't dehydrate you as much. This one is loaded with vitamins and fiber.

1 large navel orange, peeled and sectioned
$1/2$ cup iced tea
$3/4$ cup orange sorbet
3 ice cubes

Place all ingredients in a blender and whir until smooth. Makes about 3 cups.

Just Do It

So much of our energy gets bound up in indecisiveness. Should I buy the car or put the money in my retirement account? Should I get that new sofa or not? We go round and round trying to decide, and days, weeks, months pass. Then there's the energy that gets lost in regret and hindsight—I should never have bought the house. If only I'd chosen the other couch.

One way around this is to set a time limit for a regret-free decision—I will choose by Tuesday. Then figure out what you need to make the decision: more information, input from others, or whatever it is. Finally, go get what you need by the deadline and decide, knowing that you will not look back with regret. Period. If you find yourself going down the "if only" path, remind yourself of your commitment and say to yourself, "I chose the best I could with the information at hand. Now I am here. What shall I do—live with it, or decide to change it?"

A Moment to Be

We all know that meditation is "good for you." It can lessen anxiety, stress, and depression; quiet critical thoughts; free up energy; and promote concentration. So why don't we do it more? For one thing, we build an identity around being busy and productive, so we resist what seems to be just sitting and not doing. For another, the process of meditation—noticing self-criticism and resistance—isn't always as pleasant as the resulting sense we get of ourselves beyond the self-criticism and resistance.

Enlightened masters say that the purpose of meditation is beyond purpose, just to be. But until we get there, our minds need a purpose to grasp. We need an answer when our minds protest, "Why sit here when you have a stack of dirty dishes up the yinyang?" Meditation can have many purposes: Stilling the body. Taking time to notice yourself on the earth. Relaxing. Visualizing emotional or physical healing. Discovering what we believe. Becoming aware of the reality beyond our concepts. Learning to concentrate so the mind gets less disturbed by things out of our control. Touching in with God, a deeper wisdom, or higher essence. A moment just to be, not do.

If this sounds good to you, see the next entry for a way to begin.

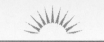

Refresh with Awareness Meditation

Meditation wasn't designed as an energy restorer, but that certainly is one of the side effects. Because it allows your brain to produce more alpha and theta waves, which are at a slower frequency than our "paying attention" beta waves, it actually restores your mind.

There are many ways to practice, but here's a typical beginner's technique. Sit comfortably in a chair with your body straight but not stiff, and your shoulders relaxed. Place your hands comfortably in your lap or on your knees. Allow your eyes slowly to close. Feel your belly gently expand and recede, rising with each in breath and falling with each out breath. Notice your body touching the chair or floor. Now become aware of your breath as it passes by the nostrils back and forth, in and out.

When thoughts arise, notice them and then let them go. If sensations appear in your body, notice them and let them go, too. Bring your attention back to your breathing each time it wanders off and simply experience each in breath as it comes into your body and each out breath as it leaves your body. Feel or imagine the breath moving through your body, down into your chest, into your belly, your legs, and your toes on each in breath. As best you can, avoid judging yourself or your thoughts or feelings. Just note them, trying not to pursue them or reject them. Return to the breath, maintaining moment-to-moment awareness as it continues to move in and out of your body.

Remember Aloud

Do you recheck the oven to be sure it's off or the door locks because you can't remember if you've locked them? A quick energy-saving tip is to say aloud: "I'm turning off the stove" or "I'm locking the door." The sound of your voice will remind you that you've completed a routine task.

Learn "Square" Breathing

Square breathing is a simple way to get the most from your breath. Talk radio psychologist Dr. Joy Browne swears by it. You can use square breathing to sidestep anxieties that drain your energy (like the what-ifs that crowd your brain while rushing to the airport), as well as simply clearing away the cobwebs when you need to focus.

Why is it called square breathing? Because you divide the breath into four parts—inhale, hold, exhale, and hold—for equal lengths of time. You do it like this: inhale (one, two, three), hold breath in (one, two, three), exhale (one, two, three), hold breath out (one, two, three). Repeat the cycle two or more times to get the best effect. Of course, longer counts help you get a fuller breath, but it's not a contest! Go gently.

This is an easy one to teach children to do. And a calm child is an energy booster, too.

You May Suffer from
Chronic Fatigue Syndrome

The Center for Disease Control estimates that 500,000 Americans are suffering from Chronic Fatigue Syndrome (CFS). CFS is a mysterious condition that has no known cause and no diagnostic lab test. Rather, it is diagnosed through a constellation of symptoms that include unexplained fatigue, joint pain without swelling or redness, muscle aches, sore throat, swollen lymph nodes, loss of short-term memory, insomnia, and headaches that can't be explained by depression, obesity, substance abuse, or other disease. For years, physicians dismissed sufferers as being depressed or hypochondriacs, but now medical science takes the condition seriously despite the wide range of severity and various combinations of symptoms.

If you are constantly exhausted for no particular reason, you should check out *www.cde.gov/ncidod/diseases/cfs* and consider seeing your doctor. Treatments vary depending on symptoms.

Go Outside

Believe it or not, being cooped up in the house can drain your energy. Research has shown that people need one half hour of natural sunlight a day to keep the brain producing the correct amount of serotonin, the feel-good hormone.

Cut Down on Alcohol

A glass of wine may make you feel less tired, but the effect is very temporary because it's a sedative—you're feeling less of everything.

Alcohol saps energy in two ways. First, it dehydrates you, which means less oxygen gets circulated in your bloodstream. Second, while it may make it easier to fall asleep, chances are you'll wake up in the middle of the night. The disruption of your brain-activity patterns linked to restorative sleep can have a bounce-back effect. So if you have three-in-the-morning wide eyes, perhaps you need to cut back on or eliminate alcohol.

Wiggle or Move as Much as Possible

When we sit in one spot for long periods of time—at computers or on airplanes, for instance—blood gets drawn away from our brains and hearts and pools in our legs. This can cause a sluggish feeling. The more you move around, the more you keep the blood circulating and your energy up. So get up, walk a bit, or at least move your feet around in circles.

Pop a Vitamin B5

According to *The Real Vitamin and Mineral Book*, vitamin B5 helps to unlock the energy in food. It is found in chicken, yogurt, and peanuts. If you want to make sure you're getting enough, you can take a supplement. The recommended dose is 100 milligrams per day.

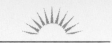

Become a Convert to Green Tea

In the past decade, more and more is being discovered about the benefits of green tea. Studies have shown that while green tea is lower in caffeine than coffee (it has only one-fourth the amount), it actually produces more physical energy. The reason is that green tea contains catechins, which activate brain chemicals to increase nerve action and their energy levels.

Use Energizing Soap

Aromatherapists have been teaching us for years that certain scents wake us up while others mellow us out by causing the brain to release various chemicals. Take advantage of this effect by showering in the morning with soap that perks you up—peppermint and citrus are particularly effective. But don't use them at night when you want to mellow out!

Try the "Breathing Machine"

Thank goodness breathing is automatic and involuntary or we'd all forget to do it. But when we add awareness to our breath, we employ a powerful energy booster that is instantly available. Adding body motions to our breathing enhances the pick-me-up even more.

Here's a simple way to breathe with motion. Face straight ahead, then inhale as you turn your head to the right, exhale as you turn back to center. Repeat for the left side. If you have more room, try this variation: Stand or sit erect with your arms at your sides. On your inhale, raise your arms out from your sides and over your head—can you feel your ribs expand? On your exhale, slowly lower your arms back to your sides.

For a twist—literally—try this: Feel your feet on the ground or bottom on the chair. Inhale as you raise your arms so your palms face each other above your head. Exhale as you move one arm straight in front and the other behind, palms toward the ground. Keep your head and hips facing straight ahead. On the inhale, bring your arms back above your head. Repeat, switching arms as you exhale. To end, let your arms slowly descend down to your sides as you exhale. A breathing machine!

ENERGY
BOOSTER

18

Remember What You Can— and Can't—Control

One reason we get so depleted is that we run around trying to control the people in our lives, which is a hopeless task. And the more we understand this, the less energy we'll expend trying.

In this book *The Inner Game of Work*, author Timothy Gallwey lays out all the factors that are not in your control in an exchange with someone: the other's attitude or receptivity; how well the other listens; the other's motivation, needs, or priorities; the other's time availability; whether the other likes you; the other's ability to understand your point; how the other interprets your communication; whether the other accepts your point or does what you want.

So what can you control? You. You control your attitude toward the other, your attitude toward listening, how receptively you listen, your acknowledgment of the other's point, your respect for the other's choice to accept or decline, your respect for other's time, your expression of enthusiasm for the other's idea, the amount of time you spend listening and speaking. Ask yourself: Whom do I need to give up trying to control to gain energy for the things that I can influence?

Mold Could Be Making You Tired

Recent studies have shown that as many as 40 percent of buildings in the United States contain mold. It is such a problem that some insurance companies around the country are refusing to issue home owner insurance because of mold. Mold doesn't just do damage to your house, but also your body: symptoms include headache, problems concentrating, rashes, mood swings, respiratory problems, and, yes, extreme fatigue.

To learn how to reduce the risk of mold in your house and how to eliminate the mold that may be there, the government has a Web site with all the details: *www.epa.gov/iaq/molds/index.html.*

ENERGY
BOOSTER

20

Go for the Good Carbs

In the past decade, nutritionists have discovered that there are two kinds of carbohydrates—those that deplete energy by creating a spike in blood glucose levels one hour after eating and then a crash, and those that increase energy by keeping blood glucose levels more even. To have sustained energy all day long, you need to eat carbohydrates with a glycemic index (GI, the measure of the rate glucose enters the bloodstream) below 70. Eating low-GI foods at night helps you sleep more soundly. And for those wishing to lose weight, there's an added benefit: eating low-GI foods helps curb cravings and snacking.

Low-GI foods include virtually all fruits, multigrain and sourdough bread, low-fat yogurt and milk, all kinds of beans, brown rice, pasta, most vegetables, and even many desserts. You can find a more complete glycemic index by looking on diabetes Web sites.

Manage Your Energy Like Your Bank Account

Energy is finite—just like money is. And we need to think about managing it as we do (or should) money. Just like money, there are three questions when it comes to energy management: How can you get more for daily use? How can you save for the future? And how can you make what you have go further?

ENERGY BOOSTER

22

What happens when you ask yourself these questions? What changes do you need to make in your life so that your day-to-day account is in balance, you are maximizing your daily expenditure, and you are saving for the future?

Restore Mental Energy with Flower Essences

Flower essences are substances created by a complex process of steeping. Herbalists swear by two for increasing the capacity to focus on mental tasks: Impatiens (*Impatiens glandulifera*) and Indian pink (*Silene californica*). The usual dose is four drops of each, under your tongue, four times a day. Flower essences are available at health food stores.

Become Aware of Breathing

You already do it. But do you notice it? Simply becoming aware of breath adds to its power to renew and refresh. Notice your breath (without changing it, if you can). Feel your stomach rise and fall. Maybe you can feel your ribs open to the back, sides, and front. You might try using your breath as an internal masseuse. Let it expand that perpetually tight spot between your shoulder blades.

Notice if you tend to breathe more into your abdomen or upper chest. Then try letting your breath extend into the part that normally doesn't get much air, to your collarbone or your belly button. Can you feel a difference? Perhaps relaxed muscles, perhaps renewed attention and calmness.

A subtle and interesting thing occurs when you pay attention to your breath. Your deeper self remembers that there's more to life than worries, tasks, feelings. That you are a vibrant human, whether or not you get everything done. Let yourself remember the wonder of being alive and breathing: that little forgettable miracle we do ten to twenty times a minute, 15,000–30,000 times a day.

Eat Spicy Food

Wake up your taste buds with some zinging flavors. Try Indian, Thai, or Chinese food (but say no to the MSG, which will have you snoozing in an hour or so). You'll get a particular lift from opposing flavors like sweet and sour—they actually stimulate the brain, making you feel more alert.

It's Okay to Be Tired

Ever notice yourself trying to bargain about being tired? "I shouldn't be so tired, it's just Tuesday!" We weigh the seven hours of sleep against the dinner to be made, meetings to be planned, homework to be supervised. "I can't be tired, I have so much to do!" Maybe we fear that admitting our tiredness will open the floodgates and we'll keel over. Actually, it's the judgments that needlessly drain energy.

See for yourself. Take just a minute, maybe when you're driving to pick up your kids or on the bus. Say to yourself, *I shouldn't be so tired*, or the related injunction, *Snap out of it*! Do you feel more alert? Or more defensive? Notice your reaction in your hands, face, breathing. Now say to yourself, *I guess I'm tired right now*. Do you collapse? If you're like many people, you feel lighter, more present.

How you approach tiredness—as a friend, a fact of life, or a foe—affects how you make it through your day. Either within your body or ten steps ahead of it dragging it along on your errands. Try acceptance for more energy.

Give a Little Smile

Smile! as a command generally doesn't work. Who wants to be told what to feel or how to express it? And the aspiring beauty queen who smiles through a car accident seems disconcerting, not inspirational. Still, it's been proven that smiling does make you feel better.

Studies in Germany have shown that people who read cartoons while smiling found them funnier. And American researchers discovered that imitating facial expressions of stress and anger caused the same physiological responses—increased heart rate and body temperature—as recalling stressful experiences. But smiling actually creates the relaxation response.

Buddhist monk Thich Nhat Hahn advises smiling during meditation—or any time. This isn't stretching your lips into a pumpkin grin. Think instead of a half smile or inner smile. Just raise the corners of your mouth slightly. See if you notice a shift in your sense of well-being. With an inner smile, you'll have more energy to handle life's stresses.

Indulge in Downtime without Guilt

We all need downtime. Plants need winter dormancy to bloom. Hedgehogs need hibernation to conserve energy. Humans need sleep to process the events of the day. Maybe you already take time to exercise or have a cup of tea or play solitaire. But if you do it while feeling guilty—always keeping one foot in the door of "shoulds"—you're erasing the rewards.

Carolyn Hax, the astute *Washington Post* advice columnist, says that berating yourself for lying on the couch instead of hitting the treadmill is "a complete waste of valuable couch time." Instead, she suggests writing "Lie on couch" on your to-do list, then crossing it off when you're done. "Sometimes," she continues, "the best way to get more done is to ask a lot less of yourself." In order to find the energy to go on, we all need to tune out on a regular basis. So turn off the "shoulds" and indulge.

ENERGY
BOOSTER

28

Acknowledge Real Body Needs

Do you eat when you're mad? Do you search the computer for an old high school friend when you really need to sleep? Do you talk on the phone when you want to exercise? (As Will Rogers said, "Whenever I feel the need for exercise, I go and lie down for half an hour until the feeling passes.") This is what you think the body wants, but not for the long term.

When you're tired, angry, trying something new, it's easy to distract yourself with the most familiar comfort you know: food, TV, cigarettes, hanging out. And it works—temporarily. But the rebound can make you feel worse. When you seek an energy boost in the wrong place, it's like trying to get a good haircut in a hardware store. It's just not there.

Changing habits takes practice. Gently and repeatedly, guide yourself out of the hardware store, over to one of the other 364 energy boosters in this book. Eventually you'll be sitting in a salon chair—acknowledging and meeting your real body needs for eating, sleeping, moving, and more.

Stay Alert in Groups

A meeting or class can create a powerful—and embarrassing—urge for a nap. To keep alert, consider what helps you to stay alert. Does it help to be able to glance out a window? Doodle? Tap your foot quietly? Stand up in the back? Take notes?

You might want what is often called the "power seat," facing the door. Even if you're not interested in power per se, seeing who's coming and going—and what mood they're in—helps you become more engaged, more energized. In a class, sitting close to the teacher might be more motivating—or at least a bigger deterrent to nodding off.

Check out the lighting and temperature in the room. Darkness, flickering fluorescent bulbs, too much heat can either make you sleepy during the meeting or sap your energy afterward. Another reason to consider a seat by the window: The natural light is easier on the eyes, and you might be able to open the window to let in a breeze if the room gets stuffy. Each of us needs something different to help stay energized. Notice what works best for you and give yourself permission to do it.

ENERGY
BOOSTER

30

Try Mind Mapping

Energy can drag when it's being siphoned off into a problem you keep trying to settle: a work proposal, an upcoming test, a wedding. Your mind goes over and over it, like a tongue over a new filling. You might use a to-do list or outline to get organized, but in order to access the most creative part of your brain, try mind mapping.

A mind map looks like a flower or branches of a tree. In the center of the paper is the circled main topic surrounded by branches of related ideas, which in turn have their own array of smaller related concepts. Using arrows, pictures, and placement, you can link and free-associate all the interrelated parts of the problem. In the end, a mind map can be used to study from or convert into a linear checklist. You can use mind maps to brainstorm large topics and then write up the mind map as a list to reflect the order in which to accomplish things. When you get the whole problem—and some solutions—on paper, it frees your mind from working it over and over. And voila—more energy!

Take Off Your Watch

Do you like to know precisely what time it is at all times—how many minutes left to eat, to read, to drive before you have to do the next item on your list? Is your watch the first thing you put on in the morning? Do you feel a little naked without it, glancing down at the moles on your left wrist for comfort and validation?

Guess what? You don't need a watch. If you look around, you'll see how easy it is to find out the time without one. All around you are clocks—in the bedroom, on cell phones, on the stove, on time-infatuated pedestrians who are only too happy to look at their watches for you. You can be bare-wristed and still as punctual as a watch wearer.

Try a day of being watch free. You may appreciate what you are doing, instead of how long it takes to do it. Or if you don't want to rely on the kindness of strangers, put a watch in your purse. It's there if you need to check it or even wear it for a couple of hours. As Dr. Andrew Weil says, "I often think of a watch as a slave band, the source of unnecessary and unhealthy stress."

Access Your Intuition

You might have a good guess as to why you are so tired. It could be obvious—especially if your child is waking several times a night. Or there might be a more subtle cause. Rather than trying to figure it all out rationally, take a moment to use your intuition to sense what's usurping your energy.

Find a place where you can have a few uninterrupted minutes. Close your eyes. Notice your breath, your body, where you make contact with the ground (your seat or the floor). Visualizing with soft eyes or an open heart, scan your physical body for pain, tension, or illness. Notice the sensations, words, colors, or how the energy vibrates in those areas. Notice the sensations of emotions. Perhaps a tearfulness behind your eyes, tension near your heart, clenching in your jaw. Now let your soft eyes or heart scan your mind: What problems is it grappling with? A rebellious teen? A lost job? Finally, see if you have a sense of yourself beyond your body, beyond your emotions, beyond your problems. A sense of being part of something bigger.

When you're ready, open your eyes and, like a computer program, "save" the sensations or images or knowledge you gained from this time. When you know where your energy is going—illness, unacknowledged emotions, thorny problems, or feelings of powerlessness—you can then take steps to remedy the energy drain.

ENERGY
BOOSTER

33

Be a Kid Again

Childhood ingrains deep memories on our neural pathways. Reconnecting with whatever made you joyful in childhood can be freeing and energizing. In autumn, jump in leaves. In winter, build a snowman or make an angel in the snow. Make pretend birds' nests from freshly mown grass. Build a sand castle at the beach. (Don't supervise it, do it!) Play "A–My Name Is Alice" or hopscotch or hide-and-go-seek. Build a Lego. Or hide in a fort.

ENERGY
BOOSTER

34

It takes energy to suppress our kidlike joy, so ignore the jealous glances from "real" grown-ups and play!

Give Bee Pollen a Try

Bee pollen is one of nature's superfoods—it contains all twenty-two amino acids, making it a complete protein, plus twenty-seven minerals; vitamins B1, B2, and B6; niacin; pantothenic acid; folic acid; vitamins C, A, and E; and enzymes and coenzymes. Herbalists recommend one to two teaspoons fresh, raw pollen a day as an energy booster; each teaspoon contains 4.8 billion pollen grains. Some folks are allergic—so take a few grains first to make sure it doesn't have adverse effects in you.

Forget Whatshisname

Can't remember the name of the music teacher your son had five years ago? Don't sweat it. Facts naturally fall out of our gray matter, young or old. The human brain has a limited capacity for remembering names. Why? Our brains evolved when most people lived in villages. Villages of, say, 150 people.

But today, our minds are cluttered with names—names of fellow committee members from ten years ago, models of Toyota cars, book titles, TV shows, Lucy Ricardo's landlord, your state legislator (you forgot?). Accept this information overload as a fact of brain function, not aging, memory loss, or lack of caring.

So save your brain power! Smile when you remember the face and be unapologetic when you ask for the name again. Don't stress about forgetting and you'll get less tired out.

It's Okay to Be Eccentric

Do you tend to be very nice? Very, very nice? Social norms help us be vital members of society, family, and workplace, and they're nothing to scoff at. But how much energy are you spending on making things just so, on fitting in rather than standing out? If you spend much of each day trying to be unruffled, or helpful, or masterful, or fulfilling any image of who you should be, try out a day of a little eccentricity.

Eccentricity is not about others noticing you or thinking you're special or weird. It's to use your own life as a creative medium. As Jack Kornfield, the Buddhist teacher says, it's "finding the freedom to be utterly one's own person." Do it for yourself, to make yourself smile. Put a plastic spider on your rearview mirror. Wear that bright red shirt your Aunt Wanda gave you. Put hairclips on your polar fleece hat. Arrange a pile of pebbles beside your porch stairs. Paint one wall of your bathroom saffron yellow.

"I hope I'm becoming more eccentric," says Tom Waits, the quite eccentric musician. "More room in the brain." And more verve in the life!

Do the Twist

Yogis believe that body twists are energy boosters. They release tension along your spine, allow more nourishment to your spinal nerves, and massage your digestive organs. The easiest twist is seated—at your desk or before you start up the car. Sit near the front edge of your chair or cross-legged on the floor. (For a deeper stretch in a chair, place your right ankle on your left knee.) Feel your "sit" bones press toward the earth and let your head float up, making space in your spine.

ENERGY BOOSTER

38

Inhale and, if you have room, open your arms out to the sides. Exhale and turn to the right. Place your left hand on your right knee or thigh, while bringing your right hand behind your back to your left hip (palm facing out). Start the twist from the base of the spine, thinking of each vertebra moving freely. Be gentle with your neck, keeping your chin pointed over your breast. Take several breaths, growing tall as you inhale, twisting slightly more as you exhale. Release the twist on an exhale. Then do the pose to the left side. Before you run off to the next thing, "save" the feeling of expansion in your body.

Build Energy with Herbs

Several herbs that you can add to your meals are reputed to replenish energy. You can grow them in your garden or find them at a health food store. They include:

Burdock root: used like carrots
Dandelion: roots added to soups and stir-fries; leaves added to salad raw or steamed
Licorice: roots steeped for a tea (not recommended for those with high blood pressure or on heart medication)
Nettles: leaves, roots, and young tops steeped as a tea with raspberry leaf

Practice Positivism

We really do have a choice to see the glass as half full rather than half empty. And when we look at what's right instead of what's wrong, we give ourselves renewed energy to face life in all of its complexity. Focusing on what's wrong—with ourselves or others, or with circumstances—drains and depresses us, depleting energy. Noticing what's right produces the uplift of hope and possibility.

This is not to say we live in denial about the problems in our lives, simply that we ask ourselves questions such as: What could be right about what's happening right now? What good might come of this? How can what's going on help me get what I want? What can I be grateful for here?

Tune Out and Turn Inward

These days we are under a great deal of pressure to pay attention to everything that is going on around and outside ourselves all the time. Cell phones, pagers, e-mail—all these so-called convenience items draw our attention outward every minute of the day. But the human brain also needs to pay attention inward—by spacing out, day dreaming, or meditating. This is how we process what happens to us so that we learn from experience and are refreshed to begin another day.

One of the reasons meditation is so popular is that it gives us a structured way to turn inward. But you can also doodle mindlessly, wander aimlessly, listen to music without words, or do whatever allows you to tune out the outside world. Try doing it for fifteen minutes a day and notice the renewed energy in your daily life.

Use Crystal Power

Crystals and gems have been used for centuries for their healing properties. Turquoise, for instance, when placed on the thymus gland, is purported to help balance and regulate energy. To give it a try, lie down and place a turquoise stone on your thymus for a few minutes. The thymus is located right below the notch in your throat. If nothing else, the rest will do you good.

Don't Try to "Catch Up" on Sleep

Sad but true—if you try to catch up on your sleep by staying in bed longer on the weekend, it can backfire and make you more tired. That's because if you change your sleep cycle by two or more hours, you upset your circadian rhythm, that inner clock that regulates your wake and sleep cycles. Your body will think it can sleep later on Monday, and you'll end up groggy all day. The more you can stay consistent with your sleeping and waking times within sixty minutes, the less tired you'll feel.

Open Those Hips

Try this simple version of a yoga hip opener when you're tired from a day in front of your computer.

Sit on the front edge of your chair, feet on the floor. Use your abdominal muscles to create a long, tall back. Let your head float upward. Place one ankle on top of the opposite knee, forming a triangle with your thighs and calf. Inhale, lengthen, and slowly lean forward and extend out in front. Lead with your heart, keeping your neck and back long. Let your arms hang down at your sides or rest on your open knee, deepening the stretch.

ENERGY
BOOSTER

44

Only go as far as the stretch permits—let your body be wherever it is today. Relax into the stretch for five or more deep breaths. On an inhale, slowly curl up one vertebra at a time. Switch legs and repeat on the other side. Aaah.

Drive for Steadiness, Not Speed

Driving is draining, especially on congested slow-and-go freeways. Highways were designed for continuous flow, but needless braking creates a domino effect of brake lights in back of it. Traffic slows and then eventually gets back up to speed.

Computer traffic models have shown that space in front of cars permits traffic to merge and flow more smoothly and may help everyone arrive a little bit faster. Would you rather drive for twenty minutes at high speed only to be stuck in a traffic jam for twenty minutes? Or at half speed for forty minutes? Driving for steadiness won't give you an adrenaline rush—and the subsequent energy drain—of keeping that tricked-out sports car from cutting in front of you. Instead, you'll get a sense of ease and relaxation.

Try an experiment during your next commute. Keep a steady speed and try to maintain at least a semi-trailer length in front. It will allow cars to merge, but you will also have an easier time merging yourself. You may not decrease your commute time, but you'll decrease the time it takes to recover from it!

Note Your Accomplishments

We do a lot each day, but it's easy to forget all that when we're hurrying to the next task: a school meeting, groceries, loading the dishwasher. And as pleasant as it would be, a coworker will not likely say, "Hey, you got that monthly billing out again! Great job!" Nor will your kids say, "Thanks for driving me to piano lessons!"

Keep a page of your journal or calendar to mark and acknowledge what you've done. When you're starting a new habit (exercising for example), put a small sticker on the calendar for each day you do it. When you've accomplished a difficult task, send a prearranged e-mail to a buddy. Acknowledgment keeps you on track and honors the person your achievements matter most to—you.

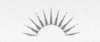

Enhance the Exercise Effect

If you're like most people, you feel pretty good right after you exercise. Blood is flowing, toxins were released in sweat, your head is clearer. You can maximize that feeling by "saving" it, just like you save a word-processing document to the computer.

Many yoga classes end with a relaxation, called *savasana*, which helps bring attention to the effects of the yoga practice. You can appreciate and save the good feeling after any type of exercise—and you don't need to lie down to do it.

Craig Mardus, in *How to Make Worry Work for You*, suggests taking twenty minutes to relax after exercise, but even three breaths enhance the exercise effect. Just take a moment before you jump into the shower to consciously experience the endorphins released in your body. Feel the blood cleansing your veins and arteries; feel your muscles—achy maybe, but stronger; feel your breath deeper and smoother; feel your mind, less ruffled and more in the present moment. Appreciate yourself for instigating the exercise and your body for its effort. Savor the energy you unleashed, and you'll find it helping you throughout the day.

Brush Your Body
as Well as Your Teeth

Getting your circulation and lymphatic systems going is not just invigorating, it's healing. You can quickly do just that before, after, or during your shower with a bath brush. The technique is attributed to a Chinese healing art called Qi Gong. The intention is to help your lymphatic system, located just beneath your skin, drain the toxins it has filtered. And it feels great.

Use a dry, long-handled bristle brush, sweep your limbs and torso toward your belly button or your heart—see which one feels better to you. Start from your feet or hands using long sweeping motions. The brushing can be continuous (e.g., toes to belly button then heels to belly) or in sections (the top and undersides of one arm, then that shoulder to belly).

From your feet, brush from toes to the top of the thigh, then over your hips and buttocks to your stomach or heart. From your hands, brush toward your shoulders, down the front of your chest, and down the back. Don't forget to include a pass over each side of the neck (lots of lymph glands here). But you'll probably want to avoid the face—the technique feels too rough. Even if you don't buy the medical perspective of cleansing your lymph system, it feels enlivening to wake your skin up in this way!

You May Be Suffering from TMS

Unless you are one of the rare few who transcend the attachment to possessions, you probably have TMS—too much stuff. Too many toys, sweaters, kitchen appliances. Too much of anything. TMS most often takes the form of clutter—piles of homeless books, magazines, catalogs, toys, cosmetics, CDs, papers, mail to be read, knickknacks, cat brushes, clothes, craft projects. Clutter drains your energy. You either avoid looking at it or you get overwhelmed with all the decisions involved in caring for or tossing each item. Clutter fills the surfaces of your home, keeping you from having the energy for the things you really want in your life.

As Marla Cilley says on her Web site *www.flylady.com*, you can't organize clutter, because most clutter consists of things you aren't sure you really want. Clutter is a pile of indecision. Before you can actually rid yourself of clutter, you need to see it for what it is, and how it's affecting your life.

A first step is to grab a grocery bag and find twenty things that are broken, unusable (like a single earring), or have no value to you or someone else (expired vitamins). Move quickly. When you've found your twenty things, throw them out. Feel good? Maybe you want to throw out even more.

Maybe You're Bored

Sometimes we're tired because we're not stimulated enough. Our lives become too routine and so our energy flags. One way to figure out if this is the cause of your tiredness is to ask yourself, Where am I being challenged in my life these days? Where am I being asked to grow, to stretch, to learn? If you can't think of anything, perhaps you need to add a bit of challenge into your life. Take a class, learn a new hobby, ask for more responsibility at work. We feel more alive when we stretch ourselves beyond our comfort zone, but not if we go into stress. The trick is to find something that is stimulating but not anxiety producing.

Figure Out If You Suffer from Food Allergies

You can develop allergies to certain foods—particularly when they are overeaten—that can leave you feeling exhausted. Common culprits are soy, wheat, corn, dairy, and nuts. Apparently what happens is that these substances don't get completely broken down and the body releases antibodies to fight these "invaders." Because you eat it so often, the body keeps putting out antibodies, which can result in fatigue as well as other symptoms such as bloating, gas, and achy joints.

To see if this is why you're feeling low, eliminate all soy, wheat, corn, dairy, and nuts for two weeks. Then add them back into your diet one at a time, while keeping track of how you feel in a food diary. If you find that one of these is causing fatigue, eliminate it completely for three to six months. Then try again, but only in moderation—once or twice a week.

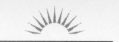

Rearrange Your Space

Recharge your senses by rearranging your home or office.
Seeing your sofa, desk, or pictures in new spots will awaken
the brain—and your creativity.

Strengthen Neck Muscles

Holding up your head is a lot of work—after all, your head weighs about fifteen pounds. And weak neck muscles can lead to headaches, neck and shoulder pain, and fatigue. Most workout routines ignore neck strengthening exercises.

Here are two simple ones. Sitting down, interlace your hands and place them at the back of your skull. Press forward with your hands while resisting with your head. Hold for three seconds. Repeat ten times. Now place the palms of your hands on your forehead. Try to press back while resisting with your head. Hold for three seconds. Repeat ten times.

If you suffer from severe neck or back pain, get professional help; doing these wrong may add to the problem.

Cut Out Emotional Energy Drains

Sometimes we feel exhausted because we're drained emotionally. In her book *The Emotional Energy Factor*, Mira Kirshenbaum
identifies eight energy drains. Do any of the emotional habits in
the list below sound like yours? If so, consider putting into action
her suggestions for breaking the cycle:

> **Other people's expectations:** Declare independence
> from what others are asking of you. If they are disap-
> pointed, that's their business.
> **Loss of self:** Find ways and places for you to be more of
> who you really are.
> **Deprivation:** Treat yourself in small ways daily and plan
> something big to look forward to.
> **Envy of others:** Practice gratitude for the good things in
> your life.
> **Worry:** Take action, if only making a to-do list.
> **Procrastination:** Pick one small thing and finish it. Or
> decide that you aren't ever going to do it and cross it off
> the list.
> **Overcommitment:** Say no to something so you can say
> yes to yourself.
> **Holding on to loss:** Cry until there are no tears left and
> you are ready to move on.

Put a Snap in Your Step with Schisandra

Schisandra is a Chinese berry that is used to increase mental and physical energy. It's available at health food stores and Chinese herbal stores in powder or capsule form. The daily dose that is recommended is 1.5 to 6 grams standardized to 9 percent schisandrins. Don't try it if you're pregnant or have a seizure disorder or high blood pressure. And stop taking it if you develop a rash, heartburn, or stomachache.

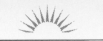

Find Homes for Your Stuff

One reason we put papers and other items aside, forming hills of clutter, is that we don't want to decide where they should live. But these mounds of unresolved problems create a subtle drain on your energy, filling your head with "where is?" and "I should."

As professional organizers will tell you, there are easy items in clutter piles—those that go to a specific room or into the recycling. And then there are things you really do have to make decisions about. When faced with these decisions, we suddenly want to—have to—take a nap, pull up dandelions, or make a four-course dinner. Don't berate yourself for having difficulty putting papers away; it does take a little focus. Think of it as an investment, one that will return energy.

Set a timer for five or more minutes and find a permanent home for seven items in your pile. Do this a few times a week, or every night before you go to bed, and soon you won't feel like you are being chased by clutter demons in your own home.

Ground While Driving

When we're overtired, we tend to lose track of our bodies, spacing out into a world of thoughts, ideas, and daydreams. This is fine if you're on the sofa, but not so good when you're driving. If you can't pull over for coffee or a five-minute nap, you can still give yourself a shot of focused energy by grounding.

Grounding is simply feeling attached to the earth, not free-floating. You can do it anywhere, even going sixty-five miles per hour in a luxury car with high-performance suspension. Just notice your thighs, bottom, and feet and how they are touching the car. Pay attention to the bumps and dips on the road, like you were reading Braille with your legs. Notice how your body leans on turns, notice your hands on the steering wheel. You might even notice the air on your skin. That should bring you back to the car, giving you the energy to get to where you're going.

Center

Being tired spaces you out: You can't absorb information, you escape in daydreams, you need a break. You can counter that spaciness and have more focus and attention if you get centered in your own body.

Most people have an intuitive sense of what centering means: connected in your body, touching the earth. Centering helps you be aware of your surroundings and sensations in your body and environment. It helps your body feel safe. When you are centered, you have a better sense of what you want and what you need.

You can use your imagination to center: Imagine a cord dropping from the base of your spine, extending down through the floor and the ground, attaching to the center of the earth. The cord can be anything: a beam of light, a root, a rope, a chain, whatever you like. You can imagine sending your tiredness, irritation, someone's judgments down the cord to be recycled at the center of the earth. And you can bring up the energy of the earth through your feet to make an energy circuit. Once you connect to the earth, you can connect to your body and have its power available for you.

ENERGY
BOOSTER
58

Give to Yourself

For a few moments, think about giving in your life. Do you give away your energy or do you hoard it? Do you give because it's necessary (making grilled cheese for your children) or because you choose to?

If you constantly give yourself away, maybe part of you believes that the emotional needs of others are more important than your own. Take a moment to answer this question: If a genie popped out of this book and said, "What emotional needs can I fill for you?" what would those needs be? The need to be noticed or to have alone time or to have engaging conversation or to be in a clean house? Pick one of those needs and make it a priority.

If you constantly hoard yourself—holing up with the Internet or work or TV—you might be unable to access a larger source of energy. So you hide from everyone's needs, including your own. Ask the genie to help you identify your deep needs and how to fill them. Maybe a walk instead of surfing the net. When you fill your needs, you have more energy, and more to share with others if you choose. Be a sweetie to yourself!

Focus on the Next Step

We're told that to be a success we need to plan our path. But we waste energy and time trying to figure out how to create the plan. Instead of worrying about all the ramifications of the possible outcomes, focus only on the next step. For instance, if a job opportunity arises, you do your best on your resume and cover letter. You don't spend too much time second-guessing how the job or lack of response might affect your life.

The next step allows your life to unfold naturally instead of following a perfect linear path. When your life unfolds, the "bad" choices are correctable and may even have positive influence later. From this unfolding place, see if there's a deeper wisdom beyond your mind—a gut instinct, a higher power—that knows the most beneficial next step. Once you trust the next step, your mind executes what needs to be done. When the next step is complete, let it go and move on to the next next step.

Sleep Better

A good night's sleep gets you rejuvenated, but it may be elusive. Check with your doctor to find out if there's a medical cause (from allergies to hyperthyroidism to menopause) or a medicinal cause (an interaction of medications, even ones that initially caused sleepiness) contributing to the problem. If not, here are some tips that may help you catch those elusive Zs.

What are your physical needs for sleep? Darkness, quiet, coolness, comfort top most people's lists. There are sleep props—eye masks, noise machines, fans, and mattress pads—that can help fill these needs. Create rituals and habits for the transition to sleep that are relaxing, soothing (not the time to start your taxes), repetitive, nonstimulating. Let yourself let go of the day, writing of gratitude, worries and peeves, or to-do lists. And if you still can't sleep, try using Calmes Forte (a homeopathic and herbal remedy recommended on *Slate.com*) for deep relaxation.

For further information, check out some of books (*The Well-Rested Woman* by Janet Kinosian or *Say Good Night to Insomnia* by Gregg D. Jacobs) and Web sites (*www.iSleepless.com*) on sleep. And if you habitually stay up late reading instead of going to bed? Close this book now. Good night!

Tap into Your Sexual Energy

They don't call it energy for nothing! It's the primal drive, the pleasure from being close, the urge to celebrate and continue life. Sex—alone or with a loved one—can relax you, energize you, put you back in your body. An executive wearing a red lace teddy under her career suit knows that this isn't necessarily about maintaining femininity but about keeping connected to a glow of aliveness and spark.

Explore your sense of your sexual body as an energy, not an act, and it can help you breeze through your day.

Put a Plant on Your Desk

A living, breathing green plant that is. Plants take in carbon dioxide and give off oxygen, so you will actually get more oxygen in the air you breathe—and that in turn will keep your mind fresh.

Expand Your Chest

This is a great yoga pose for instantly improving energy. (It gives you better posture too!) Sit cross-legged. Place one hand behind your back with elbow bent, fingers facing up toward head. Place your other arm straight over your head and then, bending at the elbow, place your hand behind your back. Try to touch fingertips together. Hold for three breaths, then release and reverse hands (if left was on top, now do right).

If you can't get your fingertips to touch, take a small towel and grasp the two ends behind your back with palms facing toward your body.

Up Your Metabolism

You are probably aware that different folks have different rates of metabolism and that affects not only how much you can eat without gaining weight, but also how much energy you have. The bad news for women? Men have a faster rate than we do, and as we age, our metabolism gets slower and slower: beginning around age twenty-five, women's metabolism slows down about 2 to 5 percent each decade. But you can increase your metabolism and thus your energy at any age by exercising more and eating right.

One key is to increase muscle mass because muscle burns 90 percent more calories than fat. Another is to not skip meals or go on extreme diets (less than 600 calories a day), which causes your metabolism to slow down to compensate for the "starvation" it is experiencing. Also make sure you get adequate protein to maintain or build muscle mass (best are egg whites, lentils, nonfat yogurt and milk, lean beef, grilled chicken breast, salmon, turkey, and tofu) and enough sleep so that you can do all that working out.

You Could Be Anemic

Dr. Ravi Thadhani, assistant professor of medicine at Harvard Medical School, says that more than ten million women are, at minimum, borderline anemic. Anemia is a condition of the blood where, due to a lack of iron, hemoglobin levels drop and the body gets less oxygen. Symptoms include fatigue, feeling cold all the time, paleness, weakness, and brittle nails. The fatigue usually comes on in the afternoon because you've depleted so much energy in the morning. To find out more, go to *www.anemia.com*.

But don't get too much of a good thing. Men and post-menopausal women often suffer from an overdose of iron, which has been linked in some studies to increased risk of heart attacks. So consult your doctor before pumping iron.

Energy Down the Drain

Do an inventory of where you are spending the majority of your emotional, mental, spiritual, and physical energy. Is this where you want to be spending each? If you are stuck in some energy-draining situation—with a person, a job, debt—what actions could you take to resolve things or change how you are relating to them?

Experience the Energy of Creativity

Spark, creative energy, divine inspiration: Even the words about the creative process describe movement, light, and power. Some say that creativity comes from beyond our thinking mind, but whatever the source, creativity can recharge our lives.

"But I'm not creative!" you moan. "I don't have the time!" Or "I don't know what to do!" Fear not. Creativity can take many forms. It can be a deep, life-changing path, or a dance class, or rearranging your furniture. A visit to a museum or botanical garden can get you started.

Your critic may tag along during your initial creative forays, wanting you to paint a Matisse on your first canvas. But you'll find the energy in the process, not the product. If you stay focused on that, you'll bring openness and relaxation to the rest of your life.

Get a Quick Energy Burst

In her *Family Herbal*, herbalist Rosemary Gladstar gives a recipe for a drink that will give you a quick spurt of energy when you need it. It's not recommended for everyday use because guarana contains caffeine, which overrides exhaustion.

> 2 packages Emergen-C®(available at health food stores)
> 1/6 tsp. guarana powder
> 1 cup water

Place in a shaker and shake until blended. Makes 1 cup.

Suffering from Sinusitis

Sinusitis is an infection of the sinuses that is caused by a bacterial infection or by constant irritation due to allergies or pollution. Symptoms include stuffy nose, headache, and fatigue, which are so similar to those of colds and allergies that it can be hard to know what's going on. That's why, although it is the most common chronic illness in the United States, millions of folks suffer in silence—they simply don't know to go for treatment. If you suspect you might be one of these silent sufferers (and your symptoms have persisted more than ten days), go to the American Academy of Allergy, Asthma, and Immunology Web site at *www.acaai.org*.

ENERGY
BOOSTER

70

Breathe from Your Belly

Ever notice how much energy kids have? It's not just that they are younger. All children know a secret to greater energy—they breathe from their bellies. Just watch a young child for a minute and you'll see—the abdomen rises and falls with the breath. This is the way we were designed to breathe.

But something happened to us all around puberty. We began breathing only from our chest, thus depriving ourselves of the invigoration a full breath gives. To do it right, sit tall. Breathe slowly in through your nose until you feel your belly expand. Then exhale slowly until your belly is flat and the air is completely out of your lungs. That's it. If you practice ten minutes a day, it will soon become automatic.

Take Vitamins at Night

You'll sleep more soundly and therefore feel less tired if you take your multivitamin at night. That's because the calcium and magnesium found in multivitamins are soporific—they help you feel sleepy. And you may want to up your dosage of these two minerals. In *Female and Forgetful*, naturopath Elisa Lottor recommends at least 500 milligrams of calcium and 250–500 milligrams of magnesium before bedtime.

ENERGY
BOOSTER

72

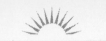

Dislodge Creative Blocks

You face a deadline for a proposal or a work project. No matter what you do, when you sit down to work, your ideas all seem recycled, stale, or—even worse—nonexistent. Trying harder just gives you a headache, but when you relax you just imagine critical comments from your boss. Like a traffic jam, everything is piling up around this bugbear: your creative flow, your energy, and the million other things you need to do.

73

Walt Disney's take on the creative process might get your project moving again. Disney had three distinct personas in his creative flow: the dreamer, the realist, and the spoiler. For creative ideas to become manifest, each persona must have a say at the proper time.

First allow yourself to dream and imagine solutions without worrying if they are doable. After the dreams have percolated awhile, let the realist in you assess whether these ideas will work within the constraints you have—budget, client needs, physics. And finally after you've made progress on your work, ask your critic to come in for what it does best—an analytical assessment of what you've done well and what you can do better. Remember the old adage, "Too many cooks spoil the broth." To keep your creative juices bubbling, invite your creative chefs into your kitchen one at a time.

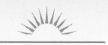

Cry, Baby

Unless you let it move, sadness—chronic or acute—can clog you up, putting perpetual tension into your eyes, heart, stomach, and lungs. Crying is not the only way to release sadness, but it's a darn good one. Research conducted by Dr. William Frey, biochemist and tear expert, showed that emotional tears differ chemically from tears caused by cutting onions, indicating that crying releases specific toxins. Even Aristotle theorized that a good cry "cleanses the mind."

How do you make yourself cry? You can sneeze when your nose tickles, cough when water goes down the wrong pipe, yawn when you're sleepy, bang pillows when you're angry, and release sexual energy when you're aroused. But letting tears flow involves opening yourself to the feelings from within.

Start by giving yourself some uninterrupted time, probably alone, since crying near others might keep you from focusing on your own experience. Watch a stirring movie, listen to ballads of longing, or read a heart-rending book. (Kids' books like *Charlotte's Web*, *The Bridge to Terabithia*, or the last chapter of *Winnie-the-Pooh* can be poignant and fast reads.) All of these can give you permission to release your sadness.

When your eyes start to water or your heart feels tingly, focus on your physical sensations. Let your thoughts—ranging from everything will be okay to it's so awful—be in the background, not dictate your feelings. Don't rush the process. Let the tears flow. Big girls—and boys—do cry.

Try a Little Night (or Day) Music

"Music hath charm to soothe the savage breast, to soften rocks or bend a knotted oak," said poet William Congreve. Music can also excite, energize, relax, and provide company for difficult or mind-numbing tasks.

When your energy sags as you're preparing dinner, put on some oldies or music with a dance beat. If you're feeling lonely when you're straightening up, let a good vocalist provide company. When thoughts of work are competing with concentrating on traffic on the homeward commute, try some Bach concertos or Handel's *Water Music*.

A subject of much research, Mozart's music has been shown to help with alertness, which is attributed to the music's tempo, sound frequency, and structured variations of melody. According to Don Campbell, author of *The Mozart Effect*, his music "helps clarify time/space perception"—which may be another way of saying it helps you stay focused on the here and now. You don't need a "soundtrack for your life," but a little musical accompaniment is an easy way to add some sparkle.

Sing

Most Americans only give themselves permission at Christmastime to do something that they deny themselves the rest of the year: sing! And not just singing, but singing with others in choral groups, choirs, and caroling.

People who sing are healthier than people who don't, according to research at the University of Surrey in Britain. Singing tones the lungs, strengthens the abdominal and intercostal muscles of the diaphragm, stimulates circulation, improves aerobic capacity, and releases muscle tension.

You don't need "holly and some mistletoe" to reap the energizing benefits of singing. Open your mouth, take a breath, let your vocal chords vibrate, listen to the sounds. Start by humming in the shower (the acoustics are great) or sing your child to sleep. Put on your coming-of-age tunes in the car and belt out "My Girl" or "Once in a Lifetime" or "The Rain in Spain." Wail along with Reba while you fold your laundry.

Can't sing, you say? Bah, humbug. Humans are born with an innate perception and understanding of music. Even Celine Dion uses amps and reverb to boost her sound. And if you're tone deaf—so what? The sacculus, a small organ in the inner ear, registers pleasure from certain frequencies emitted by singing, say researchers at the University of Manchester. So you get pleasure no matter what it sounds like to anyone else.

Loosen Your Neck Ties

Your neck does a heck of a lot of work for such a small body part. It carries your breath, your food, the nerves from the brain, spinal fluid, blood—while balancing the weight of a fifteen pound bowling ball on top. So when your neck is tense, your energy to think, breathe, balance are blocked as well.

Releasing the tension in your neck requires a gentle and steady approach. Sudden movements or ignoring pain can cause later discomfort, not release. For a simple revitalization of your neck, first sit tall with your feet on the floor. Place your elbows on the desk or table in front of you. (You can also do this pose with your elbows in the air or when you're lying down.) Drop your chin to your chest and curl your back so your fingers can reach behind your head. Gently and steadily use the pressure to lengthen not only your neck but also the tops of your shoulders. Take six to twelve breaths. Then remove your hands and uncurl your body, bringing your head up last.

ENERGY
BOOSTER

77

Boost Up with Boron

Studies by the USDA reveal that people who have a lot of boron in their bloodstreams perform better on tests of memory and concentration. And how do you get boron? Raisins are a great source—and they are so easy to carry around with you.

Give Yourself an Out

If you find yourself swamped with too much to do, you may have difficulty saying "no" to requests for your time and energy. The cause may be something simpler than guilt, habit, lack of assertiveness, or lack of boundaries. It may just be that you are taken by the present moment. (That's something we all strive for, right? How could that be a problem?)

When you're at a productive meeting, having coffee with a friend, or simply in a relaxed mood, your to-do list may fade. Sitting among friends or colleagues, it's easy to forget the soccer club fundraiser or the yard work or your resolve to have free time. You want to be helpful, so you say, "Sure, I'll design the Web site," or "Need help with the auction?" In these situations, give yourself time. Say, "I'd like to help, but I'm not sure I can fit it in. Let me get back to you."

This gives you time to check your calendar, your deepest desires, and where your priorities really lie. Then use Miss Manners' suggestions for saying no: gracefully, regretfully, and without needing to offer explanations or excuses.

Massage the "Oh No!" Spot

There's a place that will help you renew, and it's right in the middle of your forehead. Touch the flat or indented spot about an inch above your eyebrows, centered above the bridge of your nose. It's the place where you put your hand when you comfort a sick child, try to remember something, or when you say, "Oh, no!"

Many consider this spot to have power. The Hindus put a bindi (a decorative mark) here. Some call it the third eye or sixth chakra (energy point). Energy practitioners say that touching these neurovascular points keeps blood circulating in the forebrain and soothes the body's automatic stress response. Touching there generally revitalizes.

Yoga practitioners use resting the forehead for many restorative poses. A simple way is to place your hands palm down on your desk or table, one hand resting on the other and fingers pointed toward your extended elbows. Push back your chair a little and rest your "Oh No!" spot on the top of your hands. Breathe. Or place your elbow on the table and rest your forehead in the heel of your palm. Or simply hold your fingertips on your forehead. Oh, yes!

Consider an Ayurvedic Remedy

Bacopa monniera is a plant extract that has been used in India for more than three thousand years for improved mental energy, work production, and information retention. Even kids take it to do well in school. Also called Brami, after Brahma, the creator of the universe in the Hindu pantheon, this supplement is best taken in powdered extract form because of its bitter taste. Follow label instructions.

Embrace Darkness

When's the last time you were in the dark? Total darkness. Even when we sleep, the sodium street lights creep in past our curtains and create an amber dusk on the bedroom wall. The world has become if not nocturnal, at least lit. Satellite photos of Earth at night show how we live in constant brightness.

All this light affects our natural circadian rhythms and our hormones, which regulate our sleepiness and wakefulness. Darkness cues the brain's pineal gland to secrete the hormone melatonin. Melatonin seems to facilitate the onset of sleep—and may support our total health, cites the *British Journal of Cancer*. Researchers say that darkness helps create a deeper, more satisfying sleep.

Embrace a little darkness. Dim the lights as you go to sleep to help you unwind. Get some light-blocking blinds or a good quality eye mask. Turn the clock radio away from directly shining at you. Remove nightlights to only the hazardous recesses. Let the dark help you relax more fully and sleep more deeply.

Drink Some Maté

You'll find this on store shelves as a ready-made drink. Maté is made from a South American herb and is a great pick-me-up because it contains about as much caffeine as tea (about half as much as coffee). Reputedly, it is nonaddictive and won't cause sleeplessness. Loaded with nutrients, including vitamins A, C, E, B1, B2, and B-complex, plus iron, calcium, biotin, potassium, and manganese, it is said to boost the immune system, clean the blood, and stimulate the mind.

Tennis . . . Ball, Anyone?

Tension in your back is a subtle but constant drain on energy. It's like water pressure: When you're running your sink, your shower flow gets lower. Life circumstances, difficult emotions and thoughts, working at a computer, all these things create tension in your body—especially down your spine. If you don't happen to live with a massage therapist, it can be hard to rub that tension out on your own between or instead of regular massages.

But a tennis ball massage does wonders at work or any place with a high-backed chair. Sit tall, place the tennis ball alongside (not on top of) your spine or on an aching area. Lean back into it. Take long, smooth breaths.

If you find yourself tensing your shoulders, mouth, or another spot because it hurts, lessen the pressure. Or rock gently side to side. When the tension has eased a bit, move the tennis ball to another spot; you can focus on one side at a time or go for symmetry. Don't forget your lower back, and try it on your glutes (buttocks).

Hum

Humming as an energy boost? You'll be surprised at how well
it works. It's subtle enough to do sitting in your car, quietly on
the train, or at your desk (depending on how close others are
if you're in a cubicle warren).

If there's a song haunting your brain, hum it and it may dissipate. Hum a tuneless meandering melody on an exhale and
feel how the vibrations enliven your senses, your sinuses, and
your chest. Hum your sadness. Or hum the flowers blooming.
You may even envision the humming relaxing the tension out
of your neck. Humming gets you out of your rut, puts you in
harmony with all that's around you, and allows you to be part
of the larger energy of life.

Test Your Blood Pressure

Everyone wants low blood pressure, right? Well it turns out that you can have too much of a good thing. Or more specifically, some folks have a disorder called neurally mediated hypotension, which means their blood pressure falls rather than rises when they stand, exert themselves, or get overheated. This deprives the body and brain of oxygen and causes dizziness, lightheadedness, memory problems, and—fatigue. It can't be picked up by a regular blood pressure test—you need to be tested on a tilting table. For more information, go to: *www. ourfm-cfidsworld.org/html/nmh.html.*

Stretch Your Toes

Reflexologists say that tension in the body is mirrored in, and can be released through, the soles of your feet. The toes correspond to your head and face, the arch to the liver and digestive organs, and the heel to your lower back, say Barbara and Kevin Kunz, authors of *My Reflexologist Says Feet Don't Lie*.

You can find a reflexologist to work on your feet. You can buy bumpy insoles that stimulate the nerve endings as you walk. Or you can stretch your toes and feet wide anytime (works well in stupefying meetings or traffic jams) to give your whole body a lift.

Press down through the balls of your feet, pulling your toes back. Roll your ankles to the outside to stretch the arch. Lift your toes and balls off the floor to stimulate the heels. Press through the inner foot to stimulate the calves and arches. Then complete the circuit on the balls of your feet again. Wake up your feet and the rest of your body follows.

Get Rid of Negative Energy

When you've had a difficult day or an encounter with a challenging person, get rid of the negative energy you've absorbed in the experience. Stand up and put your palms together, fingertips facing down. Rub your hands together for two minutes, imagining the negative energy leaving your body through your fingertips and going into the ground. Afterward, you'll feel more positive.

Fatigue and Your Menstrual Cycle

If you feel more run down than usual after your period, you may be suffering from anemia brought on by menstruation. This is particularly common for women with fibroids that cause extra heavy bleeding. Gynecologists recommend trying a multivitamin with iron during your period (unless you should not take iron for some reason, such as constipation—iron worsens that).

Rev Up with Red

Why are stop signs and lights red? Because red jolts senses awake, say color therapists, instantly increasing energy. You can take advantage of this fact by surrounding yourself with bursts of red—flowers, a bowl of bright red apples, a red shirt. When you find yourself flagging, focus on red and get revved up.

Indulge in a Simple Pleasure

Delight Deficiency Disorder is a condition identified by Paul Pearsall, author of *The Pleasure Prescription*, that results in irritability and that worn out feeling. "When you're not getting delight in your daily diet, your body begins to starve for its spiritual nutrients." Its cause? Taking ourselves too seriously, forgetting to indulge in the simple pleasures of life. The cure? Lighten up and find healthy ways to bring pleasure back into your life. "If you don't find a balance between pressure and pleasure, your epitaph is going to read, 'Got everything done, died anyway.'"

Delight Deficiency Disorder leaves us feeling lethargic and numb to our lives. Are you suffering from DDD? You need a dose of simple pleasures. Everyone's are different—just be sure to indulge a bit.

Maybe You Need CoQ10

Coenzyme Q10 is a nutrient that boosts production of ATP, which is the molecule that fuels almost all of the body's actions. Doctors at Manchester Memorial Hospital in Connecticut have found that most people can increase their stamina and energy with a dose of 90–120 milligrams per day. To be effective, it must be taken with food because it needs fat to be absorbed properly.

ENERGY
BOOSTER

92

Check Your Adrenals

The adrenal glands produce cortisol, a stress hormone that is supposed to regulate energy by being elevated during the day and lowering at night so you can sleep. However, because of the chronic stress so many of us are under, our levels of cortisol can get so elevated that our adrenal glands go into overdrive, producing high levels of cortisol all the time and eventually creating a condition called adrenal exhaustion.

There are blood tests to determine adrenal burnout; ask your doctor. You might also want to check out *Tired of Being Tired* by Jesse Lynn Hanley, MD, and Nancy Deville, which goes into detail about symptoms and treatments.

Roll Yourself to Vitality

Your feet absorb a lot of abuse, from fashionably uncomfortable shoes to standing at work to hauling a toddler around on your hip. It's not always easy to massage your own feet to release the energy-sapping blocks stored there. But you can unleash that energy with the faithful tennis ball—resilient and just the right size for rolling away the knots.

Stand or sit so the ball is beneath your bare or stockinged foot. (Don't try to do both feet at once while you're standing, unless you have great balance or something to hold onto.) Let your body guide you—if it hurts, lighten up a little or rock and roll the ball over the tense spot.

Start by letting the ball rest under your toes, stretching them out. Then experiment with spots on the ball of your foot, the arches, the heel. (Be especially careful if you have plantar fasciitis—heel pain—or bone spurs.) Don't be too quick to move from spot to spot. Often it takes five or six breaths, or more, to allow the tension to release. And don't neglect the second foot!

Yawn

Despite recent studies, it's still a scientific mystery as to why we yawn. And why yawns are "contagious." (You're almost yawning just reading this, aren't you?) But with research showing that eleven-week-old fetuses yawn, we can assume there's some purpose. Theories on why we yawn range from physiological (low oxygen or high carbon monoxide in the blood) to evolutionary (baring teeth to synchronizing family bedtimes) to boredom (which doesn't explain why Olympic athletes yawn before their events).

But we know that yawning stretches the jaw and the back of the throat, increases oxygen consumption, releases carbon monoxide, and sometimes brings cleansing lubrication to the eyes. That's an energy boost.

Try a self-induced yawn and see if it enlivens you. Start by pretending. Yawns are catching, so pretending can create a real one. Open wide. Wider! Take a long, slow inhale; keep your mouth wide while you exhale. And soon your natural reflexes will take over. Just make sure you're not listening to your boss when you do it!

Scratch Your Hands

Reflexologists say that stimulating your hands—just like your feet—helps clear tension and congestion from the corresponding organ. Your head, brain, and sinuses correspond to your finger tips, your digestive organs to the palms, and so on. A quick way to enliven yourself is to scratch them—your hands, not your organs.

Lightly and briskly, scratch your fingernails back and forth across your whole palm, and then move up and down your fingers. Don't forget your thumb. Next scratch the backs of your hands, running from the fingertips to your wrists if you want to keep your energy within, from your wrists to your fingertips if there's energy you want to release. Be sure to switch hands. You'll feel the stimulation linger.

Consider Cordyceps

Cordyceps is a Chinese remedy for fatigue and general run-down feeling. It is actually a fungus that stimulates the liver to release glucose into the bloodstream, giving an energy surge. It also helps restore the adrenal system. It is available in capsules at health food stores; follow label instructions.

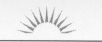

Downsize

Are you exhausted from trying to keep your lifestyle going—a big house, two cars, hot tub, wide screen TV, kids in private schools? So many of us have put ourselves under tremendous financial, mental, and emotional strain with the choices we've made. We have to work ourselves to the bone to pay for it all, and then there is all the work of upkeep and maintenance. Maybe it's time to scale back. Do you really need a 3,000-square foot house? That speed boat? The big yard?

What can or should you let go of so that you don't feel so drained all the time? Thousands of years ago, the Chinese philosopher Lao-Tzu said that the secret of life is to know when enough is enough. Where do you need to apply that to your life?

Eat More Shellfish

Eating shellfish can help you send more energy to all parts of your body. That's because shellfish of all sorts are loaded with iodine, chromium, iron, and vitamin B12. Clams are particularly good—one steamed clam contains all the iodine and vitamin B12 you need in a day! So bring on the linguine and clam sauce. But make sure to thoroughly cook all shellfish to avoid food poisoning.

Try Acupuncture

Acupuncture is an energy balancing treatment that has been used in the East for twenty-five hundred years. It is based on the understanding that your body has an energy flow, called Qi, running through it and that health problems are caused by blockages or excesses of Qi. Acupuncture has been found to be effective in treating many disorders, including fatigue.

An acupuncturist uses tiny needles to stimulate various points along the fourteen body meridians through which Qi flows. Sometimes the needles are also heated with herbs. If you want to give it a try, be sure you find someone accredited by the American Academy of Medical Acupuncturists and that they use disposable needles to prevent infection.

Have a Drink at an Oxygen Bar

Oxygen bars are springing up in big cities around the world. For a price, you breathe in 99 percent pure oxygen through plastic tubes. Some even include choice of "flavoring": mint, lemon, orange, for example. Proponents claim all kinds of health benefits of these oxygen "shots"—including renewed vitality.

Take a Ten-Minute Walk

Rather than a mid-morning or mid-afternoon coffee break, try getting up from your chair and out of the office. Walk as fast as you can and take stairs instead of the elevator.

ENERGY BOOSTER

102

Researchers at Northern Arizona State University have found that if you take only a ten-minute brisk walk a day, your fatigue will disappear for up to two hours. That's because moving increases the flow of oxygen in your bloodstream and causes the brain to release invigorating chemicals such as norepinephrine. Not only will you feel more perky, but you also will be burning extra calories!

Give Your Head a Good Scratch

People are often described as "scratching their heads" when they are trying to come up with a solution to a problem. This head-scratching cliché has a basis in physiology. Scratching brings blood flow to the brain, stimulating and soothing all the hard-working neurons.

Extend a fingertip to the base of your skull where your spine meets your head, at the indentation between the two long splenius muscles running down your neck. Scratch lightly to stimulate the spinal nerves that connect to the brain. Scratch each temple and trace an arc just outside your ears.

For the full-deal head-scratch, just dance your fingertips all over your skull. Or run your fingers in parallel furrows from your forehead and temple to the base of your skull. (To the casual observer, this just looks like you're keeping the hair out of your face.)

Revitalize without Sleep

Everyone gets insomnia at one time or another, but some of us have long-standing dates with sleeplessness. It may be our natural predispositions or instigated by PMS, medications, stress, caffeine, or environmental factors. Insomnia can rob us of our energy—if we let it. But even when all the tricks to sleep through the night fail and we still find ourselves tossing and turning at two a.m., we can revitalize without sleep.

The trick is to view the night as a time of renewal, led by the body. Not a time of busyness led by the mind. Think of it as free therapy or personal-growth time. Keep the lights off or low. When your mind spins on plans or worries, write them down along with your deepest wisdom about why they're bothering you. Then find a way to focus on your body. It could be your breath, or a progressive relaxing from toes to head, or a visualization about the tension in a particularly stubborn area. Keep coming back to your body; tell your mind that you'll catch up with it in the morning. Imagine letting a caring person hold your concerns for you while you rest. Don't worry about sleep; just rest where you are.

Even minus a few hours of sleep, you'll find you can greet the morning with a smile.

Yank Your Ears

Like a lot of personal mannerisms, pulling on your ears has stimulating benefits based on acupuncture and craniosacral massage. It stimulates acupressure points on meridians that connect to the rest of your body. Pulling on your ears can also open clogged Eustachian tubes and loosen the subtle interplay of cranialsacral bones in your head, according to some craniosacral therapists.

And it's a great way to help yourself and your kids wake in the mornings.

Gently tug all around the ears and the lobes, pulling along the natural lines of the ear. (For example, pull up at the top, back at the sides, and down at the lobes.) Certain areas of your ears will feel less pinched if you hold the cartilage closer to the center, rather than the edges. You can do this very softly and still have good results.

Maybe now you can hear yourself think!

Maybe You're Sleeping Too Much

While most of us are sleep deprived, some of us are tired because we're spending too much time in bed. So says Dr. John Shepard of the Mayo Sleep Center. What happens is this—each of us has a certain amount of sleep our bodies need. Let's say it's seven and a half hours. Once you reach that point, your mind/body begins to come awake. If you stay in bed past that point, you are working hard at being asleep, which lowers your blood pressure, making you feel weak and tired.

To find out how much sleep you really need, experiment for one week with different times. Begin with nine and cut back one half hour each day until you feel the most refreshed when you wake up.

Your Shoes Too Tight?

If your shoes don't fit right, your feet can get tired—and that can make the rest of you feel lousy too. And make sure they not only are the right size but also provide adequate padding. Shoes are basically shock absorbers. If they don't provide the right cushioning, your knees, back, and hips get the brunt of your movement, which can cause fatigue. Buy shoes in the afternoon, after your feet have already begun to swell from standing. And don't wear high heels for more than two to three hours at a time unless you want pooped-out tootsies.

Flap Your Jaws

With gum, that is. And make it peppermint. Studies have found that chewing peppermint gum stimulates the same part of the brain that wakes you up in the morning.

Load up on Tomatoes

It turns out that tomatoes are high in lycopene, which is an antioxidant that helps you feel alert and energized. Lycopene is present in all forms of tomatoes, but if you get most of your tomato intake from pizza and pasta sauce, you may be adding a lot of energy-draining carbohydrates to your diet. So take your tomatoes raw whenever possible.

What Gives You Energy?

For each of us, certain people, places, and activities inspire and energize us. The more we know what those are, the more we can choose to bring those into our lives. Take a few moments to write a list of the things—people, places, circumstances—that give you a boost, make you feel more alive. Then be sure to incorporate them into your week.

ENERGY
BOOSTER

110

I'll Scratch Your Back If . . .

Back scratching has been long ignored as an invigorating technique—overtaken by massage methods such as Swedish, Rolfing, Hellerwork, Trager, and more. But a simple back scratch (remember how good it felt when your mother did it?) can work wonders to enliven you.

Many drugstores and Asian shops sell back scratchers of bamboo or plastic. But a little cooperative arrangement can bring out the best in two people. Some like a soft scratch, some like it hard where you leave marks. Some like both, usually the soft first. Scratching works on the outside of clothes, but it's fantastic on bare skin.

Use the fingernails and a little bit of fingertips. Try "nips"—a claw-hand that scratches on the closing—or "fairy dust"—soothing, softer S curves with just a little nail.

And if you like having it done on your back, don't stop there: the backs of legs and arms are ripe for the scratching!

Hug Yourself

Here's a hands-free massage that will stimulate your muscles, your nerve endings, your sense of yourself in your body. Hug yourself. You don't have to wrap your arms around your chest (although that's a good upper-back stretch), just hug your muscles to your bones. To do this, you contract your muscles slightly to embrace your bones. Start with your feet and work up. You can hug and release one area at a time or expand from your feet to your full body. Feel your calf muscles hug your tibiae, your quadriceps contract into your femurs, your abdominal muscles massage your intestines, your latimus dorsae cuddle your ribs, your trapezius pull down your spine, your facial muscles embrace your face. Nice to have a body, isn't it?

Wake Up Refreshed

Two flower essences, available at health food stores, are known to help you wake up feeling perky. One is self-heal (*Prunella vulgaris*) and the other is morning glory (*Ipomoea purpurea*). These are remedies made by steeping flowers in water. The dose for each is four drops under your tongue when you go to sleep and as soon as you open your eyes in the morning.

Soften Your Eyes

We work our eyes hard in this world—TV, computer screens, dashboards and traffic, nutritional values in fine print. . . . Weary eyes make us feel sleepy and tired. And we can't always take a break to rest them or do eye exercises to enliven them.

We use both the rods (nighttime) and cones (normal light) to see. In daylight, the cones rely on sharp, focal-point vision as well as light from the sides, the periphery. This peripheral vision helps us balance and sense motion and shapes—it's essential for driving. Stimulating peripheral vision is good for computer work and other close work—and it's easy.

Imagine your eyes softening. See how wide you can see on the side. Play with seeing from the back of your eyes. You'll find your eye muscles relaxing, your field of vision opening, your whole face softening. You can take in more of your world with soft eyes without expending so much energy to do so.

Stand Up for Yourself

Mothers proverbially badger their kids to stand up straight. But tall bodies (no matter the height) are efficient and energizing. An erect posture is a balanced one. It allows more room for fully inflated lungs to bring oxygen to your cells and keeps your heart open to what life has to offer.

An erect posture is not necessarily the exaggerated military pose—chin tucked, shoulders thrown back, rigid body—but you can take a few cues from that pose to find your own posture center. Start by drawing your chin back—gently. Bring your head back to balance on your spine. Let your shoulders—especially the scapular bones in the back—be drawn toward your spine and down. Use your deep abdominal muscles to keep the bowl of your pelvis level; for most of us that means letting the pubic bones rise. Feel yourself growing from your feet: erect, yet flexible and powerful, like a tree or growing plant. Imagine you have a strong back and soft heart. When you stand within yourself, you have more energy.

Notice Your Energy Field

According to energy practitioner Donna Eden, energy is a language your body speaks, one that you can learn to speak as well. In fact, our bodies are surrounded by energy in a field. Most of us are just not aware of it, and the logical mind has a hard time fully embracing this, even though Einstein proved that mass is energy.

Here's how to experience your own energy: Simply rub your hands together briskly for about twenty seconds. Then bring your hands, palms facing, about six inches apart. Close your eyes and notice if you feel the energy emanating from your hands. Separate your hands or bring them closer and see where you can sense the energy and where you can no longer do so. If you can't feel any energy, either try it another time or let it go. If you want to play with it further, imagine you can see or sense the energy in your entire body, as if, as Eden says, it were a "cascading fountain" or series of lattices. Where do you most easily sense it? Where is it stuck or numb? Does your energy feel different at home, at work, at your mother's house? Once you know your wiring, you'll know where to plug in to generate more. Read on.

ENERGY
BOOSTER

116

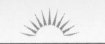

Enhance the Flow

Meridians are energy pathways in the body identified by the ancient Chinese medical art of acupuncture. Recent research using electromagnetic resistance, radioactive isotopes, and infrared photography has verified that something happens on those energy pathways that is different from what happens elsewhere in the body.

For Donna Eden, author of *Energy Medicine*, a primary avenue for health and flow is the energy in the "central governing vessel." The central meridian that works to circulate energy through all of the other channels. Its natural flow runs up your front (from pubic bone to the lower lip) and up the back (from the tailbone over the top of your head to the upper lip). To keep energy flowing in the right direction, put the fingertips of one hand on your navel and the other fingertips on the spot in the center of your forehead, an inch or so above and between your eyebrows. Push up slightly and breathe.

Even if you are skeptical about energy meridians, this simple move feels good to do, especially when you're feeling drained by external circumstances. It helps you come back to yourself. If you're in a meeting or don't want people to ask what the heck you're doing, just visualize yourself doing it.

Rock

Make the most of a relaxing moment in a rocking chair! This simple piece of furniture has been shown to both stimulate and relax, enhancing the nervous and musculature systems.

The act of rocking subtly stimulates your back, thigh, and stomach muscles. It eases depression with "kinetic therapy" according to the Medical College of Virginia. And it gently stimulates the fluid of the inner ear, which some studies suggest increases alertness. The rocking motion nourishes the cells of your spinal discs. And rocking creates an overall cellular and visceral stimulation, according to the British Medical Journal. In both babies and adults, rocking increases cardiac output and is helpful to the circulation. Gives "Rock the night away" a whole new meaning.

Pop a Pumpkin Seed

Our bodies need magnesium to create ATP, which is the molecule that provides energy to all our cells. It is found in vegetables and whole grains, but one of the best sources is pumpkin seeds. Researchers found that when women took 2.5 ounces a day, 89 percent reported much more energy. So munch away!

Shrug

Sometimes we all feel like we carry the weight of the world—on our shoulders. We fret about things out of our current control. We can't make someone healthy, can't sit with our kid as he takes the SAT, can't clean the kitchen floor when we're at work. And that fretting ends up raising our shoulders higher and higher, keeping our energy from being used on the problems we can fix, right in front of us.

With relaxed shoulders, daily stresses will slide off your back. But with tight shoulders, the flow of blood and oxygen to the brain becomes obstructed. For some, our shoulders are so tight, it seems it would take a three-hour massage to make a dent. But you can shrug off some of the tension with this version of a yoga pose.

Start by sitting tall. Exhale all the air from your lungs. Take a slow inhale as you pull your shoulders up to your ears (relax your neck and jaw as you do it). Hold for a count of two or ten—whatever feels right. Then drop your shoulders, just drop them, as you exhale with a sigh. As you do, imagine you're letting go of what you don't need and can't change. Let serenity replace frenzy.

Use the Herb the Siberians Swear By

Siberia is home to the largest forest in the world, which contains over two thousand medicinal plants. One that is great for energy is *Rhodiola rosea*, or golden root. Siberians take it to give themselves increased stamina in the bitter cold winters. According to *Natural Health Magazine*, "In one double-blind, placebo-controlled study, night-shift physicians who took rhodiola for two weeks felt 50 percent less fatigued than those who took a placebo. For same-day relief of acute stress or fatigue, take 600 milligrams of root extract capsules, divided into three doses, with meals. To continue the boost, take 200 milligrams a day on a cycle of four months on, two weeks off. Rhodiola has few side effects; however, it may raise blood pressure and could interact with blood thinning medications like Coumadin (warfarin). Do not take it if you're pregnant or nursing."

If you can't find it at the local health food store, call Yellow Emperor Herbs at 877-485-6664.

Open Your Heart

Often our chests and lungs and heart feel numb or frozen, from stress in the modern world, computer work, sadness we've not let heal. When we slump or are rigid in our chests, we prevent ourselves from making the best use of our natural energy.

Bringing energy to our chest area—opening up—means activating new feelings and muscles. You can do some simple physical chest opening right at your desk and help create support for a more open heart.

Let the inner edges of your wing-bones on your upper back—your scapulae—pull toward each other and down. Simultaneously, feel the muscles across your chest open. You'll probably notice using your abdomen and rib muscles to support yourself; they're effective and underused muscles glad to step into their role. Experiment with the image of breathing through your heart. Let your heart be open with where you are: the modern world, your work, lingering sadness. You'll find power within it.

Perk Up with Vinegar

Guess what the first sign of a tired liver is? Overall low energy. To wake up your liver and get it working well again, add more vinegar to your diet—in salads, on steamed vegetables, or by eating more pickles. Vinegar helps the liver improve its functioning by manufacturing more bile.

Try On a Lion Face

Here's a great yoga energy release, but you'll want to do it alone or among sympathetic friends. It releases frustration and tension in your face, jaw, eyes, and lungs. And it's pretty fun to do with kids!

Take a deep breath, and on the exhale do several things simultaneously: Open your eyes and mouth wide, looking at a point about a foot from the end of your nose and sticking your tongue out and down as far as it will go. Exhale firmly with sound, letting the sound come from your lungs (as in aaahhhhgggghh), not a throat scream. Let the tension and power radiate from your eyes and mouth.

Do this two or three times, taking one or more breaths between each one. Soon you'll claim the energy of a lion!

Walk to Deal with Time Change

When the time changes in the late fall, we may love getting an "extra" hour to straighten the house, party, or sleep. But the switch to standard time in the United States means we lose our after-work light and our time bearings for a day or more.

ENERGY
BOOSTER

125

The twice-yearly disruption in natural circadian rhythms prompts a temporary drop in adult alertness and function, according to the director of the sleep and alertness clinic at Toronto Western Hospital. Even when we've adjusted to the time change, the impact of darkness lingers.

Being aware of how the switch to standard time affects you will help make the transition smoother. Both these first few weeks and all winter especially in the northern latitudes, take a short daily walk outside each day. Like adjusting to jet lag, natural light will help your body. You can bounce back from the "fall back."

Have Your Thyroid Checked

We look to our busyness, our sleep habits, our stresses to pinpoint why we lack energy, but sometimes it's right under our chins: our thyroid glands. An underactive thyroid gland (hypothyroidism) will slow your whole metabolism down. According to the Thyroid Foundation of America, there are 7.5 million cases of hypothyroidism, but only a fifth of them are being diagnosed and treated.

Symptoms of hypothyroidism include cold, fatigue, memory problems, muscle cramps, depression, weight gain, constipation, and dry skin and hair. Subtle but debilitating problems, especially taken together. The treatment is a synthetic thyroid hormone or iodine-rich foods. If you think you may have a slow thyroid, see your doctor. Your energy level will thank you.

Air Out at Home and Work

We live and work increasingly in well-insulated buildings. That keeps us warmer, energy costs lower, and outside sounds softer. But it keeps fresh air out of our lungs as well. Older buildings have more ventilation, with air seeping around windows, between floors, and up chimneys. In an old house, we may be chilled but invigorated.

If you find your energy sagging—either in a meeting or on a more chronic basis, try cracking a window. Install a ventilation fan in your house or apartment. (Some building codes now require a vent fan to automatically turn on and off for a period of time each day.) Open a window at night while you sleep—your local hardware store can help you find lock solutions for windows left ajar. All that oxygen, earth, and water-fed air will help you stay peppy and alert—as well as healthy.

Take a New Route

Bored with the same old routine? Take a new route to work or to the grocery store. Your body and mind will wake up as you notice different houses, shops, plants, even the latest construction. You might even find a new restaurant to visit.

Let There Be Light

Light is energy we need to live—for food, to see, to grow. Some people are like photosensitive plants—they wilt without sufficient light. They become moody, lethargic, crabby, sad during the darker months. For those diagnosed with Seasonal Affective Disorder (SAD), light boxes, dawn simulators, southern vacations, or antidepressant medication can help.

For the rest of us, the need for light is more subtle but still significant. Simple things to keep light in our lives can make a difference. Have sufficient work light in the kitchen, at your desk, in your workshop, by your reading chair. Make sure you have ambient lighting around the computer and TV screens.

But the best source of light is outside your window. Working near a window is great, but better yet, go outside. Bask in whatever light is available—pure, without glass between you and the sun—at least five minutes a day. That might mean parking your car a little farther (you get the boost of exercise to boot) or pulling a few weeds. But your body and circadian rhythms will notice. Let the sun shine in!

Blossom!

Why do flowers make us feel better? Is it something beyond the buttery yellow of azaleas, the vibrant coral of zinnias? Beyond the round and teardrop shapes, the curved stamens, the sweet or fruity scents? What is it that draws us to follow the path of the bees to get closer to pink cherry blossoms or the purple irises?

Perhaps flowers strike us as the essence of the life cycle. Perhaps being around flowers makes that blossoming resonate within us. Whatever the reason, flowers enliven us. Bring some flowers indoors, to your desk, your bedside, your kitchen. Buy some primroses, freesia, or a flowering orchid. Bring a branch of buds from your apple tree or forsythia and watch the heat and light of your house force them to bloom. Let flowers germinate your life.

Exercise Your Eyes

It's not polite to stare, but we do it all the time. At the TV, computer screens, books, traffic. And staring is tiring, especially when your eyes become fixated and overfocused.

Flexible eyes work better than fixated eyes. A simple energizer is to remember to look into the distance—down the hall, out a window, or at a picture of a landscape—every twenty minutes when reading, working on the computer, or watching TV.

Another way to reclaim your eyes' flexibility is to do a focus exercise. Hold your finger near your nose as close as you can focus on it. Then look beyond your finger at a point in the distance. Do this five or ten times. Flexible focus means you can receive and respond to the world around you.

Start a Fire

In these modern days, we don't need fire for heat, cooking, light, safety—or even romance. But it's an essential element that rejuvenates us deep in our psyches and bodies. Fires give us the full spectrum of light with continual change and variation, the sounds of released sap or cracking wood, the transformation of logs to ashes, and the glowing architecture of the embers.

ENERGY
BOOSTER

132

The darkness of winter highlights our thirst for fire. You can quench that thirst at a gas fireplace in a restaurant, bookstore, or home. You can get it in candles placed on an intimate dining table. Or with a synthetic log—or rows of candles—in your fireplace. Or you can go whole hog with seasoned wood on a fireplace grate, fire pokers, and log turners for an evening of flames and glowing embers.

Are Your Yin and Yang in Balance?

Chinese medicine identifies two kinds of energy—yang, which is the energy associated with the masculine and is focused, directive, active; and yin, associated with the feminine, which is subtle, receptive, yielding, receding, diffuse. Are you too receptive and passive and therefore need more yang? Or are you too much of a powerhouse—assertive, aggressive—and need more yin? When we become aware of which energy we tend to rely on, we can intentionally begin to use the other as well. Rev up or become more laid back? Until you spend time analyzing your energy habits, you won't know which tack you need to take.

Slow Down Your Eating

We get more than just energy from food. We get nourishment of our eyes, our palates, our fingers, our tongues—even our nostrils when we eat spicy foods. But we miss the bounty of this energy boost when we rush from one bite to another, either from busyness, habit, or trying to dilute or distract our emotions with food.

We can tell ourselves, "Slow down!" but it helps to have a focus as we practice a new way to eat. You can buy a device that lights up or hums to cue the next bite. Or you can use your body to create your own cues.

Concentrate on noticing (look, smell, and taste) every morsel. Count to ten between each bite. Put the food or fork down between each bite. Take a minute to notice your fingers and hands; by paying attention to the periphery of your body, you expand beyond the intensity of the food in your mouth. All these ways help you remember your whole body and why you're eating in the first place.

Bundle Up in Winter

Being cold makes us lose energy. Staying warm in winter is especially important for women, whose physiology—less muscle mass, smaller frames, smaller blood vessels—often means cold hands and feet.

You'll stay warmer if you keep the heat in your central core—from your pelvic area to the top of your head. Wear layers. Keep polyester, silk, or wool close to your body to keep moisture from cooling you down. Try a thick liner glove inside your mittens. Wear extra socks or insoles. Protect your skin with the oil base in a good moisturizer.

Stay hydrated, because you can lose a lot of fluid when the cold air you inhale is drier than the warm air you exhale. Drink liquids like tea and water, since alcohol and caffeine can dehydrate you. When in doubt, drink tea with a loved one by the fire—wearing polypropylene layers, moisturizer, and a hat!

Experiment with Alternate-Nostril Breathing

The millennium-old tradition of yoga uses breathing to stimulate and enliven the whole brain and body. The yogis consider alternate-nostril breathing to be one of the best techniques to calm the mind and the nervous system. Some scientific studies have supported the concept, finding there is a natural human cycle of alternate-nostril breathing that may affect the brain hemispheres and our thinking.

In the yoga practice of alternate-nostril breathing, you bring in breath through one nostril, release it through the other nostril, then reverse. Here's how: Sit or lie comfortably. Fold down the index and middle fingers of one hand. Exhale the air from your lungs. Closing your right nostril with your thumb, breathe in smoothly to a count of five through your left nostril. Close your left nostril with your ring finger, simultaneously release your thumb, and exhale through your right nostril for a count of five. Then reverse the process.

Do three or more complete cycles using whatever count allows for comfortable, long, smooth breaths. (Sometimes you can do this with a stuffy nose or cold, but don't force it.) Many yoga practitioners add a count of holding the inhale before exhaling. After you have completed your cycles of breathing, drop your hand and take three breaths with both nostrils. Do you notice a difference?

Try an Eye Pillow

Would a short foray into deep, relaxed darkness bring you back into your own energy source? Many yoga centers offer eye pillows to facilitate deep relaxation during the end-of-practice resting pose. But you can use eye pillows any time.

Eye pillows—usually small silk or velvet rectangles filled with flax seed and sometimes dried lavender—are available at natural food stores, crafts fairs, yoga supply stores, and on the Internet.

You use an eye pillow just as you might think—lie down and rest it across your eyes. The soft silk, the gentle weight, the soothing scent, the enveloping darkness send you quickly to a restful place where you can find yourself again.

Laugh

What did the Zen master say to the hot dog vendor? Make me one with everything.

It's a rusty joke by now, but it—or another old saw—can still bring a smile to your lips. Humor has the power to break us out of our ruts, to make us see things in a new light, to encourage exhalation, to create community. Garrison Keillor, writer and host of *A Prairie Home Companion*, says, "Laughter is what proves our humanity, and the ability to give a terrific party is a sign of true class."

So how do you lighten up? Listen to Keillor's annual joke show; watch the Marx Brothers' *Duck Soup*; read the cartoons in the daily paper, alternative weekly, or *The New Yorker*; laugh at the kids' messy rooms or when you wobble attempting a headstand in yoga class.

ENERGY
BOOSTER

138

Do the Spinal Rock

The spinal rock—or spinal roll, but that sounds like a sushi dish—is done by yoga practitioners to "wake up the spine." It massages the back and neck, and helps your cerebral spinal fluid move into your brain.

Do the spinal rock on a padded carpet or exercise mat to protect your vertebrae. Start by sitting with your knees up, head bent down, and your arms wrapped around your legs. Rock backward, keeping your spine rounded. Your legs will naturally extend at the "top" of the rock and bend as you rise to sit, helping you keep a smooth momentum—like a rocking chair. Keep moving or you'll find yourself stuck.

Do the rock four to six times. Take a moment to "save" the feeling of stimulation.

Get into Your Skin

When you're frenetic from planning, reacting, talking, and thinking, tuning into your body sensations gives you a mini-break. Then you can come back to the tasks at hand refreshed.

Take a journey into your own skin. Close your eyes (if you can—if not, soften your focus). Scan your body for the first place you notice touch. Your thighs on the chair? Your feet in your shoes? Perhaps you can feel your socks. Or you notice your glasses resting on the bridge of your nose and your ears. Can you feel your lips touching? The clothes on your skin? What about the air on your skin, ruffling the hairs on your face and arms.

Through your skin, you are able to experience your environment directly. You might have the sense that the environment is embracing you as you move through life.

Take a Sabbath Day

Modern people often see the Sabbath as an old-fashioned, use-less ritual of proscription and prohibition—tight shoes, tight tie, no alcohol, no fun. But the Sabbath is being rediscovered as a one-day vacation, a respite that renews.

In the Jewish tradition, the time from Friday sundown to Saturday sundown is one where restrictions lead to freedoms—no work (including no writing), no handling money, no driving. Instead it's a day of reading, walking, connecting to your essence or God.

You don't have to be Jewish to make at least one of your weekend days special. Try honoring one day a week for a month (to make it a habit). Maybe it's a day for a special walk in the park, or a day you don't shop or work or do laundry. Or spend an hour reading or going to a place of worship.

It's amazing how simply naming a time for yourself becomes refreshing and energizing, acknowledging and hon-oring the cycle of the weeks, of the seasons, of you.

How About a Nice Nap?

Do you think that being grown up means sleeping only at night and leaving naps for toddlers and the elderly? Naps have been shown to improve alertness and cognitive performance. If you're sagging mid-afternoon, try to arrange a mininap—even if, like a wired preschooler, you just rest your eyes and body for a few minutes.

Some people disavow napping because they wake up groggy or it makes it harder to sleep at night. But napping has a different effect when you do it for less than thirty minutes and wake at least four hours before bedtime. When you first start mininaps, set a timer or alarm, or arrange someone to make sure you wake in twenty minutes (the phase of deep sleep starts after thirty minutes, which is when it's more difficult to wake). Until you're used to it, you might try napping in a place different than your bed, or with your curtains open. After you've been at it for a while, you will likely be able to train yourself to wake up after a short snooze.

Switch to Full-Spectrum Light

Artificial light can be a subtle drain on energy. Flickering fluorescents with a greenish cast, dim yellowish incandescents, even halogens can produce glare. You can see this in photographs but may not notice the everyday effect.

Full-spectrum bulbs or fluorescents provide a larger range of light. They can make the colors in a room seem brighter and peppier. And, according to some full-spectrum bulb manufacturers, they stimulate the rods and cones in our eyes and make it easier to focus. Try a full-spectrum light (available at health-conscious stores, some hardware stores, and over the Internet) in your reading lamp or dining room. Especially in winter, your eyes may appreciate getting the maximum light energy frequencies available.

Try Ginseng

Sagging energy is such an epidemic that many unscrupulous hawkers will try to sell you the latest herb or tonic for it. Some of these are useless, and some—like bitter orange—prove to be dangerous. To help you sort the hype from the help, check with a reliable source such as Dr. Andrew Weil, author of *Eight Weeks to Optimum Health* and founder and director of the Program in Integrative Medicine at the University of Arizona's Health Sciences Center.

On his Web site, *www.drweil.com*, Dr. Weil suggests trying ginseng if you need an energy boost. When ginseng is taken on a regular basis, he says, it can increase energy, vitality, and sexual vigor, and it provides resistance to all kinds of stress. He recommends capsules or a tincture of American ginseng, since the Oriental variety can raise blood pressure. The potency varies, so he cautions users to check the dosage on the product. And don't take it without talking to your doctor if you have depression or high blood pressure.

Space Out for Ten Minutes

It's a paradox, but sometimes spacing out is the best way to "be here now" and to gain the energy of your deeper self. It's worth a try when you can't get moving on your plans, no matter how many admonitions, goals, rewards, punishments you set for yourself. It might be time to take a deliberate break.

Even when you're clear about your goals and feelings, the mind needs time to process, says therapist Ragini Michaels, author of *Facticity: A Door to Mental Health and Beyond*. And sometimes you are so full of awareness and growth, you can't absorb any more.

If you have a tendency to procrastination, this can seem like the ultimate excuse. But if you embrace your space-out needs for a finite period, you might find that you can then move on. Try using a timer for ten minutes while you zone out. When it rings, make sure you put your zone-out object away. With a clear break, you'll likely have more momentum for what needs to be done.

Have Some Sunflower Seeds

Certain rituals requiring rhythm, concentration, and stimulation give a boost. They come in many forms, including . . . eating sunflower seeds!

One woman I know swears by them, especially for driving long distances. She says, "You pick one up, crack it, pop the seed in your mouth, chew it, take the shell and dispose of it, then start again." The constant awareness and activity—plus the salty stimulation and the protein—keep her going. So much so that her family teases her about her car ashtray, perpetually filled to the brim with shells. But she gets where she's going, attentive and alert.

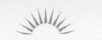

Remember the Serenity Prayer

The Serenity Prayer is: "God, grant me the courage to change the things I can, the serenity to accept the things I can't, and the wisdom to know the difference." Attributed to the theologian Dr. Rheinhold Niebuhr, it addresses the lifelong dilemma of disentangling control from influence. When we confuse the two, we waste lots of our energy on things we cannot change.

For instance, we have influence over whether we get a promotion or keep our job in a downsizing, but control only over how we ourselves perform our jobs. When we try to control things we can really only at best influence, we pour our energy down a bottomless hole. We obsess about what we might have said or done to make things different. Instead, by focusing on doing the best job you can and letting go of the outcome you can't control, you'll have more energy to do what really can make a difference.

Take a Cold Shower

A cold shower might cool a young man's ardor, but it can excite your own neurons as well. Some people swear by a three-minute cold shower to wake them up. But even just a cool rinse at the end of a bath, shower, or hair wash at the salon can provide invigorating benefits.

ENERGY
BOOSTER

148

The cold water brings blood to the capillaries, increasing circulation. Some say it reduces blood pressure on internal organs, contracts the muscles to eliminate toxins, and strengthens the mucous membranes and immune system. Even if the health benefits are not all they're purported to be, a cold shower or rinse will make your face glow and stimulate you.

Use Memory Aids

You hop into your car, sure that you'll remember the four things you need at the hardware store: light bulbs, caulking gun, picture hanger, and a new house key. But by the time you wend through the displays of halogen, fluorescent, and long-life bulbs plus ten types of caulk, you can't remember what you're forgetting.

Ideas, things to do, or things to remember pop up at the most inopportune times: the shower, on the freeway, falling asleep. Trying to keep them corralled in your brain can clog your concentration and mental energy. Use mnemonics to boost your brain power.

Mnemonics are imaginative associations—a phrase, rhyme, acronym, or image—that help you remember things. School kids learn the colors of the rainbow as ROY G. BIV, starting with red and orange, then ending with indigo and violet. There are as many ways to make mnemonics as there are to be creative. For the hardware list, you can note you have to remember four things, then picture the digit 1 screwed into a lamp socket, a 2 printed on a caulking gun, a 3 in a picture frame, and a 4 on your key ring. Or you can create a phrase from the words or initials of the items. (I caulked the picture of the light bulb with my key.)

ENERGY
BOOSTER

149

Create a Launch Pad

It takes a lot of energy to look for what you need before you leave the house—especially if you're stressing about being late. But it's easier if you have a "launch pad" by your door.

A launch pad is the place where keys, homework, briefcases, lunch, projects, signed school papers wait for deployment. It works best if you have one for each member of your family. Launch pads can be as simple as an inbox from an office-supply store, a half of a bookshelf, or waist-high coat hooks from which you hang book bags, purses, and cases off the tangle on the floor. You can add key hooks and labels, but don't waste your energy on making it perfect before you start using it.

ENERGY
BOOSTER

150

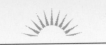

Decide to Not Decide

There are lots of ways to make a decision: weighing pros and cons, talking to friends, flipping a coin, I Ching, Ouija board, intuition.

But sometimes, a decision won't come. You replay the possibilities over and over, like a kid working a loose tooth. You make, remake, regret, or waver over which store to shop in, which music teacher to pick for your son, or whether to quit your job. The thoughts and possibilities crowd your drive home; you argue with yourself, you miss parts of conversations, you imagine telling people what you've decided.

Consider that it may not be the time for the decision to be hatched. Give yourself time to not decide. It could be just five minutes as you walk to your car, or a month, or until your birthday. It doesn't mean you won't think about it—especially if it's a life-changing scenario. It doesn't even mean you won't think "Aha! I know exactly what to do!" It means that you give yourself time for your thoughts and feelings to flow, without attaching significance to them. You have "Aha!" but you keep it to yourself for a while, telling yourself you don't have to know yet, and things may change.

You may find that when the decision is ready to be made, your answer will come from an unexpected source, and that conserving your decision energy helps you be more sure when it does.

Consider the Payoff for
Being Tired All the Time

Sure, you want more energy—you think of all you could accomplish and how much better your life would be. But what if there's a hidden reason to not having all the energy you want? When you tune into your deeper wisdom, you may discover that a part of you benefits from your lethargy.

It could be you use your tiredness as an excuse so you are able to say "no." Or you're afraid that if you succeed in life you'll leave someone behind. Or you don't want to face that you made a disappointing job or love choice.

You can harness the power and energy in these hidden objections, one step at a time. First acknowledge that the objections originally served a useful purpose. (You may have been shamed for saying no, or you weren't ready to face your decisions.) Then identify some resources to address the objection in new ways (such as saying, "I'll check my calendar," or career counseling.) When you honor the rewards of low energy, you can reclaim more of your rightful life.

ENERGY
BOOSTER

152

Put On Your Shoes

People often feel more capable, structured, professional, and energetic when they wear shoes, according to Marla Cilley, author of *Sink Reflections*. That's why many direct sales companies require their working-from-home employees to be fully and professionally dressed when making telephone calls; it makes them more effective even though the customer can't see them. But even if you work outside the home, Cilley suggests that you wear shoes while performing your morning tasks. Try it for a week and see if you don't feel more accomplished.

Fast Twelve Hours a Day

Going to bed with a full, heavy stomach can cause insomnia, restless sleep, heartburn, and may keep your food from being fully digested. All of these can deplete your energy reserves. (And some say that undigested food turns more easily into fat.)

Conversely, we can gain energy by fasting for twelve hours a day, says naturopath Emily Kane. Digestion and elimination use one third of our total energy intake each day, Kane says, and our natural body rhythms work best when our digestion rests for twelve hours. Ayurvedic medicine practitioners and yogis also suggest eliminating heavy meals three to five hours before bedtime.

An easy way to develop this habit is to set a time, maybe eight at night, and eat nothing after that. After a few days, you may discover that less is more.

ENERGY
BOOSTER

154

Wake to Music

How you wake up can set the mood and drive for the whole day. From informational NPR radio to AM radio disc jockeys to a jazzy scat by Ella Fitzgerald, waking to the right sounds can get you off on the right foot.

If you can't find a radio station that suits you, check out a CD alarm clock. Then you can wake to your favorite musician, the sounds of the ocean, or even to a customized CD (made on your computer) to start softly and build in volume.

When you honor yourself in the morning, you are more ready to take on the day.

Wash Your Eyes

Tired eyes, eyes trying hard to keep pollution out, eyes straining at work—when our eyes get dirty or tired, it's hard to keep going. That's when washing out the accumulation of pollution and strain will clear the fog. You can use commercial eye drops. Beware of overusing ones with tetrahydrazoline to clear up redness. According to Dr. Andrew Weil, they can create a rebound effect from overuse.

Many prefer an eyewash. Use a neutral boric acid eyewash like Collyrium or a freshly made saline solution ($\frac{1}{4}$ teaspoon salt dissolved in 1 cup warm water—it should taste like tears). Rinse the eye cup—available at pharmacies—with very warm water. Fill half the cup with the eye-wash solution, hold the cup tightly against one eye, and tilt your head backward. Open your eyelid wide and roll your eyeball around to let the solution wash out all the accumulated grime. Lean forward before you remove the cup, and then rinse it with very warm water before doing the second eye. We live in such a visual world, you'll find that seeing better helps you move better through your day.

Get Specific

Maybe you remember when you were a child and couldn't figure out how to clean the mess in your room, so you played instead. Then you got called lazy. It may seem obvious now how to put toys away, but you still can't think straight about cleaning the bathroom or paying bills. "Lazy" is a judgment we too often use when we mean "overwhelmed." And that judgment keeps us from solving the problem. Being specific—breaking a problem into baby steps—gets our focus and accomplishment back on track

Take a paper and list ten things that you must do to get the task done. Baby steps. For paying bills, the first item might be "make a list." (That way you'll know you'll have a success right off the bat.) The next item, find the bills; then put the bills in one place; then find the checkbook. The last item might be revising this list into a routine.

Then set a timer for fifteen minutes and start the first task—the most logical or easiest to get going. Then do the next task on the list. If you get distracted by a more perfect way to do the job, just write your ideas down for next time and keep going. When the timer rings, assess where you are. Are you ready for another fifteen-minute round? Need to revise your list? Need to set a date to continue? Whatever the outcome, celebrate it. And banish "lazy" from your vocabulary.

Note It to Others

We spend a lot of energy repeating the same things to our kids (and often our spouses and coworkers): "Clean your room. Practice piano. Remember your lunch. Don't forget the meeting with John." It's frustrating to waste your breath feeling unheard or unacknowledged.

Writing notes can be an efficient way to communicate. They're different than the usual verbal reminders, being visual. Even when kids can't read well yet, they thrill at seeing important words written for them. Teens have the distance they need to take in what parents want. And, as somebody once said, "notes don't get louder."

Stick a note on the TV, the dog, around your own neck to get the message across.

Get a Headset

In the days before telephones and televisions, neighbors would visit while one or both folded laundry, canned fruit, built a new bookcase. They had the support of companionship while they did their chores and hobbies. But in our compartmentalized modern lives, we feel thinly spread between time for friends, making supper, vacuuming the floors. We multitask at work—filing while a coworker drops by—but it's harder at home.

Technology can help in the form of cordless phones and headsets. Hands free, you can catch up with friends while you match socks, or wait on "hold" while you do a load of dishes. Plus you avoid the neck-crunching energy drain of cradling the phone between your shoulder and ear.

Most cordless phones already have a built-in jack and belt-clip, so you'll probably need just a headset to put you in a whole new mind-set about keeping in touch and keeping up.

Enlist the Neighbors

It takes a lot of energy to plan and execute a big project—moving, building a deck, painting a room, cleaning out a closet. But many hands do indeed make the task—and your heart—lighter. Bartering with friends, family, and neighbors makes the job easier and builds a net of community.

You can "chore share" informally; suggest to a friend that you help each other on dreaded tasks. Or you can make a formal co-op system where you use poker chips or an account book to log hour-for-hour trades among families.

The help of friends will mean you will likely get the task done more quickly—more focused and with less distraction—even including the time you spend returning the favor. And you can catch up with friends while you're entertained and accomplishing.

Now about that barn raising . . .

Turn Off All Beepers, Pagers, and Cell Phones

Technology is great: Knowing that you (or your teen or your spouse) can call your cell phone in an emergency eases worries. Chatting with a friend while waiting for the kids at soccer, checking voice mail while stuck at a traffic light, calling to check what's in the pantry before making two trips to the store—all of these tie busy lives together and make your life more efficient.

But technology is also a burden. The nearly unlimited cell plans tempt us to stay open, in constant touch, available to family, coworkers, bosses, and friends. The subtle but continuous availability wears us thin.

There is a simple solution. Turn off your phone. Not just at concerts or a yoga class. Pick a day of the week or time of day, and just turn it off. It's the time to prioritize being available—to yourself.

Honor Your Body's Rhythm

Your body has an inner rhythm, inner tides. In studies of people left to their own sense of time in caves or artificially lit spaces, they naturally created a twenty-five-hour cycle of sleep and waking (called a circadian rhythm). This circadian rhythm coincides with the tide cycles of twelve and a half hours, and in fact in several languages, there is a single word meaning both "time" and "tide."

While you can't live at a twenty-five-hour cycle in a twenty-four-hour world for very long, you can honor and tap into the sense of body rhythm by maintaining a regular routine. This means going to bed and waking at pretty much the same time each day.

Once your body expects a regular rhythm of sleep and exertion, it will more easily provide you with the energy you need when you need it.

Pull Your Future toward You

What words do you use to describe your life—how you spend time and energy, what you accomplish, your sense of purpose? Are you building toward your goals, cutting a path, making something happen? Notice these images all involve words of effort. What happens if you flip or shift the image? Instead of pushing toward your goal, imagine being pulled toward it. Takes less energy that way, doesn't it?

To deepen the experience of what you're being pulled toward, meet your future self. During a quiet moment, imagine being transported on a beam of color or sound to a time ten to twenty years into the future. See where your future self lives. Enter the home of your future self and see the surroundings and the person you're drawn to become. Listen to the words your future self says to you, feel the presence of the wisdom you've gained. Perhaps your future self has a name or a gift for today.

When you come back to the present moment, contemplate what you can bring into your life that reminds you of your future self—a picture, a ring, a toy. Then let that future self draw you to it.

Just Step Away

If you've ever completed a difficult crossword puzzle, you'll know this phenomenon: An entire section leaves you completely stumped no matter how many times you replay the clues. Then you look away for a moment—maybe to pet your cat—and when you look back, the answers start popping clearly into your mind. Why was that so hard? you wonder.

It wasn't hard once your brain could get a new perspective. It's the same for other stubborn problems as well: a dissertation, a piece of computer code, a letter to an old flame, the organization of your files. When you step away from the conundrum, you tap into your peripheral mental vision. Just like you can see better at night with the sides of your eyes, you can solve problems when you come back with a new perspective.

It often requires less than thirty seconds to stretch, go to the bathroom, or file a paper. Then you return with a mother lode of solutions that move your life along.

Brush Your Teeth

Here's a simple refreshing boost: Brush your teeth. Taste the peppermint or spearmint or cinnamon or bubble gum. Brush your tongue to wake the taste buds and the acupressure meridians. Stimulate your gums and smooth your teeth.

Feel like it's morning again!

Rewind Fear

Fear is exhausting. Some people describe fear as very fast energy—your thoughts and your body are jumping way ahead. Your primitive brain takes over and you hold your breath, your pulse races, your heart palpitates, you feel weak and fatigued.

In its place, fear is a useful emotion and can alert us to real danger. But when we can't get away from needless fear, we lose resources for the rest of our lives. We're overstimulated with fear in TV commercials and news, in many movies and newspapers. But we add to it by envisioning terrifying events and imagining the worst. Why? To feel like we are prepared, forewarned, in control of every possibility, says Ragini Michaels, author of *Facticity*.

To take back your life from fear, you need to say "enough" to your mind's desire to control everything. Michaels suggests that you take reasonable precautions in your life and that you address your fears by seeing them as a movie running in your head. As soon as you notice unbidden fearful scenes arising, imagine the projectionist rapidly rewinding the reel—all the movements are backward, you hear the gibberish of voices going backward. Then picture the universal sign for "No" (a red circle and slash) across the movie. Say to yourself, "That is one possible future. Not the only one." Change the sensation in your body by creating the picture or story of the future you do want. Then reclaim your life.

Dance

Dancing frees up our spirits, our bodies, our minds, and our hearts. It's an innate urge, but we stop ourselves from dancing by being self-conscious. If this is true for you, try doing it when no one else is home, or just close your eyes.

Put on some funk, pop, rock, disco, jazz, rhythm and blues, rag, swing. Feel your body from the inside and invite yourself to move as the music moves you. If you get stuck or bored, invite a particular part of your body to dance—your spine or your shoulders or the energy of your heart. Have a pas de deux with your hips. Or see what dancing would be like if you were a giant, graceful marionette. Soon you'll be saying—like Donald O'Connor in *Singing in the Rain*—Gotta dance!

Don't Let the Tank Run Dry

When you wait until you're running on fumes to fill up, you lose energy from your life. This is as true for you as it is for your car. But let's start with the car. When your gas gauge shows half empty, start thinking about a good time to fill your tank. Then you'll have plenty of time to visit the gas station at your leisure, not when you're frantic that you'll be stranded by an empty tank. Once you get in the habit, you can even schedule a particular day to fill up—every Wednesday on your way home from the gym, say. One less thing to clutter your thinking.

The habit works for other things in your life as well. The Dalai Lama says to practice meditation when you don't need it, so the habit will be there when you do. An empty stomach can make even the simplest of tasks monumental. Sleep deprivation can make ordinary irritations take on high drama. Delaying taking care of yourself can make you sick. Keep your life smooth and your energy flowing by replenishing your stock of life's necessities.

Mono-Task

Humans are so efficient, aren't we? We check e-mail and write reports during telephone conference calls. Or we shave and talk on the phone while driving. It's a boon and a bane. Sometimes we get so caught up in multitasking we get less done. Or what we do accomplish is done less well. Or we don't know where to start. We stand in the middle of the living room turning in circles, not knowing what to do first or trying to do several things at the same time.

There's value in mono-tasking. Especially when faced with a complex, distracting, or overwhelming task like sorting through the backlog of papers that need attention. Set a timer for fifteen minutes and do just one thing for that time. Just file every paper you can and make piles for others. Don't call to follow up (put the paper in the follow-up pile), don't read the magazines you haven't gotten to (tear out stories or put them in the to-be-read pile). Let the voice mail answer the phone. Stick to your mono-task until the timer chimes. Then take in the accomplishment and know you haven't wasted your time spinning in circles.

Prepare to Get Dressed

A frazzled morning can frazzle your day; you can spend hours tucking in loose ends left from a hectic beginning. The minimal amount of planning needed to smooth a morning more than pays for itself. (An ounce of prevention is worth a pound of cure.)

Tonight, before you go to bed, put out the clothes you will wear tomorrow. The earrings, scarf, tie, underwear, socks, and shoes. Then in the morning, you can let your mind and body catch up to being awake without scurrying all over looking for what you need.

A smoother takeoff for a smoother flight.

Build a Support Network

Humans, for the most part, live best in tribes—in modern life our tribe may consist of family, friends, professionals, neighbors, business or school associates, fellow joggers. A recent study showed that isolated people created an imaginary support network of TV personalities. But real people provide the boost of love, companionship, and feedback. Think of it as social sonar that can provide feedback or motivation to keep life moving forward, not spinning in a rut.

Do something today to strengthen or enlarge your support system. Find a new doctor, therapist, or car mechanic. Or ask someone to be your sounding board on a thorny problem. Or send a note thanking someone who has supported you. Knowing the ways we are not alone makes us feel safer and more able to make the impact we want on the world.

Close Your Ears

Most of us live in a noisy world. Cars, boom boxes, lawn mowers, TVs, trucks, radios, leaf blowers, planes, kids ... Some people crave stimulation and keep the talk radio on while they program or cook. Others crave silence.

Even if we do our best to tune it out, invasive or extraneous noise can invoke hearing loss, stress, high blood pressure, sleep loss, distraction, and lost productivity. It also reduces the quality of life and opportunities for tranquility.

When you can't "close your ears" but need a noise break, try earplugs, noise-reduction headsets, or white noise. White noise combines sounds of all different frequencies together, so that a single frequency—like someone's snoring—is less distinguishable. You can turn on a fan, buy a "sound conditioning" machine, turn on static on your radio, or try a CD with recordings of the ocean, a waterfall, or even a dishwasher (see *www.sleepmachines.com* or *www.purewhitenoise.com*).

Create Routines, Not Ruts

A lot of creative types think routines are chafing. But routines offer a structure, which can free creativity. Start building routines with small steps. Pick a time of day and a task and turn it into a ritual—like cleaning the kitchen sink before bed or charging your cell phone when you come home in the evening. Experts say that it takes at least twenty-one days to make a habit, so commit (and mark your calendar) to the routine for three weeks. When the routines are automatic, it unleashes your ability to make more from your life.

Do Something Right Away

Being tired creates a vicious cycle. In the never ending quest for time for yourself, you leave things for later: the toilet paper on the stairs, the library books by your bed, the dirty socks in the bathroom. Soon the house is full of little things to be done, and you feel more overwhelmed and fried—needing more time for yourself.

But doing small things as you go keeps you from having to notice or remember to do them later. And it keeps chaos from snowballing to a blizzard of stuff to do. Pick up the sock when you see it rather than waiting for the big clean up. Put the library books by the door to go back.

You don't have to do it all right away. But doing something keeps the energy flowing in your house.

Create Some Motivation

When you are motivated to do something, the energy comes from a deeply powerful place. A place of clarity, of purpose, of ease. Does motivation just happen or can it be cultivated? You can apply what already motivates you to areas of your life where you need a push.

Notice how you use your thoughts and imagination to achieve, say, a healthful running routine. Do you picture it—or taste or sense or hear words of satisfaction—about how great you'll feel afterwards? Do you schedule it in your PDA, date book, or mental calendar? Do you lay out your exercise clothes the night before or put them on first thing in the morning?

Transfer those thoughts and images to paying the bills. Picture—or taste or sense or hear words of satisfaction—about how great you'll feel with the bills paid or creditors contacted. Schedule a time to do it, and tell someone about it if that helps make the scheduling more tangible. Set up the bills, checkbook, pens, and telephone the night before. You have within you solutions that work for you. You just have to transfer your thinking.

ENERGY
BOOSTER

175

Take a Restorative Bath

Bathing rejuvenates. We let go of gravity, and our worries are diluted in the water. With a few tricks, however, the power of a tub soak is multiplied.

Add a half cup or more of baking soda or one to two cups of Epsom salts to the tub. Light candles or dim the lights to relax your eyes and face. Let yourself melt into the warmth of the tub. (Waterproof tub pillows add a special comfort.) Rest your thumbs on your temples and your fingers above your eyebrows for a few long breaths. Relax the base of your neck with a cross-hand massage—rubbing your left side with your right fingers and then the other side. Release pent-up tension in your feet by massaging between your metatarsals (long bones) toward your ankles.

Finally, if your room is warm enough, enjoy letting the water—and any worries—drain out while you stay in the tub. Slowly reenter the gravity of the earth with your energy restored.

Do a Home Energy Check

Whether or not you believe in the rules and formulations of Feng Shui—the Chinese art of placing objects to affect energy flow in an environment—you've probably experienced differences upon entering various places. A new place that immediately feels like home versus one where you can't quite get comfortable.

Take a minute to experience the energy—or simply pretend you can—of the place you are right now or a place where you spend a lot of time. Imagine that the doors and windows let in not only light and breezes, but something your mind can't quite fathom: energy. Imagine this energy flows like water; you don't want to be stuck in a stagnant eddy, nor do you want to be sitting in the rapids. Imagine what it might feel like if you moved a chair, table, or bed. Would the addition of a mirror or object you love redirect the flow?

Try using your deeper wisdom to figure out how to arrange your environment to provide you with the most support, comfort, and positive flow.

Change Mealtimes at Time Switch

Do you slump when the time changes every six months? Your circadian rhythms can get all messed up with just that one hour change. So can your liver, which keeps time as well, and regulates energy uptake from food. When the change from daylight savings time to standard occurs, eat one half hour earlier on the Friday before the time change. Then another half hour earlier on Saturday. When Sunday rolls around, eat at your normal times; your liver will now be adjusted. When the time goes from standard to daylight savings, reverse the process and eat one half hour later on the Friday before and another half hour later on Saturday.

Are You Having Fun Yet?

Often we're tired because we've had our nose to the grindstone for too long. Our mind is pooped out from all the work we're asking it to do. If your life seems like one long to-do list, you need to find a way to put more fun in your day. What do you love to do? Swim? Garden? Walk in nature? Go out dancing? When you do something you love, you engage your natural enthusiasm and thus feel more alive. And if you can't think of something enjoyable to do, that just proves how much you need it. Ask a friend to help rescue you from busyness with some fun escapade.

Tap Away Fear

Once it gets going, fear can take on a life of its own, draining our ability to think and act clearly. "If I'm this scared, there must be something horrible to be afraid of," says our inner logic.

Just as fear takes hold of the body, we can use the body to loosen the hold. Many energy practitioners suggest tapping the back of your hand between the metacarpal bones of your pinky and ring fingers, about halfway between your wrist bone and first knuckles. Tap for a minute or so. Regular breathing helps. If you still feel anxious, tap the same spot on the other hand. This may have the effect of lessening the feeling or increasing your distance from whatever is causing it, letting you get off the fear treadmill.

Tension Headache Be Gone

Tension headaches can be persistent visitors once they move in. They zap energy in several ways. The pain itself distracts or worries us. And the tension in the neck and shoulders constricts the flow of blood and cerebral spinal fluid to and from the brain.

For millennia, Asian medicine has used pressure on certain body points to effectively ease headache pain. Author of *Energy Medicine* Donna Eden suggests this routine the next time a headache ambushes you.

Massage the indents on the neck below the back of the skull. They're on either side of the muscles that parallel the spine. Make small circles along the bony ridge of the base of the skull. Move your fingers down your spine to massage the bottom of your neck. Drag your fingertips across the sides of your neck and over the front of the shoulders. Repeat the neck massage a notch higher. Continue up to the top of your neck.

Take Off Your Shoes

Just about everyone's feet swell during the day, making shoes feel tighter and cramping your energy. Some people swear by changing into casual shoes, slippers, or going barefoot when they come home.

One mom who comes home to make dinner, help with homework, and do cleaning says taking off her shoes gives her "three or four more hours." It's relaxing, it honors the transition to home, and it feels good.

You may not have time to put your feet up, but you can at least feel them wiggle.

ENERGY
BOOSTER

182

Massage Away Tension in Your Face

Smiling through your tears. Grinning and bearing it. We hold a lot of life's tension in our faces. Releasing it not only enlivens us, it lets our beauty shine through.

To release tension, massage your fingertips upward along your cheekbones. Then slowly push outward along them to your ears. Play with the location of your fingers and the pressure so it's enlivening, not painful. Try a brief rub of your temples, then down to your jaw muscles, relaxing the eyes and the mouth.

A little color in your cheeks can look good, too.

Pull Your Shoulder

Shoulders can get so tense they turn numb. Numb or achy, they still block energy between your head and your torso. A quick way to enliven our shoulders is to do a shoulder pull.

Place your right hand on your left shoulder. Apply pressure and drag your fingers forward over the shoulder. You can also move slightly outward as you do this, if that feels more relaxing. Do this pull several times before you switch to the right shoulder.

Some people, when they've done a massage, like to rub their hands together or whisk their fingers—like shaking the tension off.

ENERGY
BOOSTER

184

Pretend You're Horseback Riding

When you've been sitting for long periods, your spine and organs tend to collapse into each other. Revitalize with this supported "horse-riding stance," which will elongate your spine.

Stand with your feet wider than your hips. Bend your knees like you are sitting in a chair, and place your palms low on your thighs. Straighten your elbows and feel your spine lengthen. (You might find more support with your fingers pointed inward.) Make sure your feet are directly below your knees and pointed at the same angle as your thighs. Keeping your chin tucked, slowly twist one shoulder toward the opposite knee. Come back to center, and then repeat on the other side.

From center, let your arms hang, and then slowly roll upright, keeping your head hanging until the last moment.

Cross Your Wiring

Most people know that the left hemisphere of the brain controls the right side of the body, and vice versa. When infants crawl, they are ingraining this pattern that allows us to read, learn, and move with vigor.

When you're dragging, scrambled, or even fearful, some tasks that reinforce this crossover pattern may help you. As you walk, swing your hand across your body toward the opposite leg. Or as you sit, briskly lift your knees one at a time and touch them with the opposite hand. Try crossing your arms and placing them around your shoulders (a good upper-back stretch as a bonus). Play piano, or do pat-a-cake with a kid. Swim. Using both hands together, make sideways figure eights. Or sway your hips in a figure eight.

Anything that speeds up the cross flow of information between your body and brain will speed your energy up as well.

Turn Upside Down

Symbolically as well as physically, yoga values the experience of heart over head. Thus most yoga classes offer some inversion pose during each class. Inversions can be stimulating or restful, but by reversing the usual pull of gravity, they reliably give a sense of renewal.

A simple, restorative inversion is to put your legs up a wall. Place a bolster—a folded blanket or firm pillow (two to five inches in height)—a few inches from a wall or closed door. Then position yourself with your upper hips and lower back on the pillow, your bottom in the space between the pillow and the wall, and your legs running straight up along the wall.

Adjust yourself so you're comfortable and relax into the floor. Open your arms out to a forty-five-degree angle in a "goalpost" shape (upper arms out to the sides, forearms at a right angle pointing up). If your hamstrings feel tight, bend your knees slightly, or turn the legs slightly in, or move the bolster further away from the wall. Feel your chest open. Let gravity and your breath drain the tension out of your feet, legs, groin, abdomen, chest, arms, and head.

Enjoy this pose as long as you'd like. When you're done, bend your knees, lower your legs, and roll over on one side. Take a few breaths in this curled position. Then slowly, using your hands as support and keeping your head heavy until the end, push yourself into a seated position.

Flick It

An experience with a rude teller or an arrogant driver or your own faux pas can cloud you with anger, fear, or critical thoughts. Without noticing it, your shoulders notch higher, your teeth set, you curl a little to protect your core.

    Instead of carrying the weight of that with you, flick it out. With your arms at your sides, flick your fingernails with your thumb. Let the sneers, fears, honking, or judgments roll down your arms and be cast off. Give it to the earth to handle. Come back into your full sense of power and energy.

Ride a Roller Coaster

Are you reeling from a bad breakup? Fuming about a missed promotion? Frustrated by a snarling teen? Repressed emotions can smother your vitality, but you probably have good reasons for not having it out with your former lover, your boss, or your fourteen-year-old.

Go express your anger and reclaim your vitality and sense of humor at the nearby amusement park. Scream your fears on the falls of the roller coaster. Bash your imaginary boss at the bumper cars. Connect with your strength at the batting cage. Sail into the future at the driving range. If you're going to be angry, might as well be happy about it!

Practice to Be Imperfect

Are you pooped from perfectionism? Intellectually, you may know you're striving for an impossible goal, but emotionally, it's become embedded in your identity. You think if you try hard enough and follow all the rules, everything will go right, everyone will love you. Ah, if that were only possible!

Reclaim yourself and your humanness, in other words, your imperfections. Start by noticing your inner perfectionist: the gender, voice, dress, props. This will help you notice—and appreciate—who you are without the ever unattainable finish line. Then make some mistakes, on purpose or by accident. At least once per day. Celebrate them! Say "Ta-da!" when you notice one. Reframe mistakes as feedback (a means of learning) rather than failure (your identity).

What wonderful mistake did you make today? Ta-da!

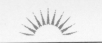

Strengthen Your Abdominals

When you tap into your core strength, you gain access to deeper and more efficient resources. This is true not only for your core values and self, but also for your physical body. When the core is weak, you overuse the peripheral muscles—trying to milk out more than they were meant to handle, creating knots and blocks.

Abdominal exercises are not just for looking trim in a bathing suit. They invigorate and enliven your core, your breath, your sense of power. They help you maintain good posture and get more oxygen in your lungs.

To start working these muscles, lie on your back, knees bent, hands clasped behind your neck. Inhale deeply and press your back into the floor as you tilt the pelvis upward. Exhale and lift your chest and shoulder blades off the floor slightly (keeping your neck long and supported by your hands). Draw your lower abdominal muscles in toward the spine and contract the muscles. Hold the position. Inhale, either returning your chest to the floor or staying lifted. Then do four to eight more cycles. Always take it slow, keeping your lower back long, your pelvis tucked, your shoulders and neck relaxed. Even if you can't lie down right now, just contract these muscles and reconnect with your power.

Bike!

Remember hopping your two-wheeler as a kid, streamers flying, bulb horn honking, or bell tinkling as you took wing through the neighborhood? It wasn't exercise or transportation—it was exhilaration.

Adulthood is no excuse to keep your bike gathering dust in the garage or keep you from borrowing or renting one. You don't have to make an expedition to rural roads or bike paths to gain the vitality of riding. Just jump on the bike. Circle the block for a quick pick-me-up. Cycle to the store for a loaf of bread or your prescription.

Whether it's the balance, the motion, the circular exercise, or the wind in your face, the great and freeing feeling of cycling will invigorate your summer days.

ENERGY
BOOSTER

192

Step Back into Your Own Eyes

When you consider your life, whose perspective are you seeing it from? Do you see yourself through the eyes of a neighbor, your older sister, a parent, a boss, your spouse?

What happens when you experience your life from behind your own eyes? You might experience a shift—owning your own power in a new way. Creating energy from aligning with your own values and criteria.

When you find yourself scrambling to meet "shoulds," shift back into your own perspective. Imagine seeing with your own eyes, hearing your own true voice, stepping into your own path, or turning a hand mirror back to see your own reflection.

Behind your own eyes, you have the answers and values you need.

Hydrate

We were nurtured as embryos in the amniotic fluid of the womb, and we die if we're without water for longer than five days. Water comprises up to 70 percent of the body and is crucial in body temperature, energy metabolism, digestion, circulation, excretion, and cardiovascular stress. Water helps rid the body of toxins, reduces sodium buildup, relieves constipation and headaches, maintains muscle tone.

On average, we need the equivalent of eight eight-ounce glasses of water a day, some of which we get from fruits and vegetables. But thirst seems to be an elusive sensation, less persistent or jarring than hunger pangs. So it's easy to delay drinking what we really need. (Go get a glass of water to drink while you finish reading this.) It's daunting to be faced with four glasses of water at dinnertime and spend the evening peeing.

Some tips to help your hydration: Keep water handy. Add a squeeze of lemon to liven the taste. Remember that a gulp equals about an ounce, so a short quench at the water fountain can equal a whole glass. Keep this essential element flowing in your body.

Create a Wheel of Life

Where does your life give you energy and where does it require more than you get back? A good way to figure that out is the wheel of life.

Draw a large circle and slice it like a pie into eight or more wedges. (This is not a science or art project, so aim for good-enough, not perfection.) Label each wedge with an aspect of your life—such as career, money, health, friends and family, significant relationship, personal growth, creativity, and fun/recreation. Then color in each wedge from the center point outward, approximating how much fulfillment you have in each area. The wheel might now look like a small circle, telling you there's room to expand in all directions. Or you may be seeing an oval shape or a flat tire.

Choose one area to work on that either needs bolstering or one that simply draws you. Write down three strategies—make them baby steps or huge leaps if you're ready—that would help you become more fulfilled in that area. Commit to a friend when you will do at least one of those actions.

Why is balance an energy booster? It's physics: The bigger and rounder the wheel, the less force you have to exert to move it.

Perk Up with Aromatherapy

When you think of aromatherapy does it bring to mind a Victorian-style perfume factory—lace doilies and olfactory overload? It can actually be a subtle and powerful way to energize your life.

The sense of smell is central to humans. It is the first sense to activate after birth, and newborns can differentiate their mother from other lactating women just by smell. Researchers are now investigating the power of scents to reduce stress and invigorate. For instance, smelling nutmeg can lower stress-related blood pressure. And researchers at the Sloan Kettering Cancer Center discovered that the floral aroma of heliotropin lessened the anxiety of MRI patients.

Being mindful of the fact that some scents can trigger migraines and allergic reactions in others, you can spice up your life subtly. Keep a tin of dried lavender or rosemary at your desk for a pick-me-up. Lavender is said to be calming, relaxing, and balancing; rosemary good for overcoming mental fatigue. Or dab some specially scented creams or essential oils (available in natural food stores) on your temples. Or invest in an aromatherapy atomizer to fill the room.

Commit Out Loud

Maybe joining an aerobics class, writing your resume, or saving fifty dollars per week will really be a great next step. But you can't seem to actually accomplish it. Knowing what to do in order to move forward in your life is no guarantee you'll actually do it.

When you verbalize your commitment—to a supportive friend or a life coach or therapist—you amplify your power to act. The listener acts as a witness to your intention and your accomplishment, not someone to shame or nag.

Be specific and realistic in what you will achieve, when you will do it, and how you will let your witness know—by phone, e-mail, in person—when you've attained it.

Just the act of speaking your intention can fill you with focus, purpose, and energy. Now imagine how you'll feel when you actually do it!

Clean Up

It sounds like an oxymoron: When you're pooped out, what might just pep you up is cleaning. Some folks swear cleaning is an energy boost. "I find that a messy house zaps me of energy," says one woman. "And the act of cleaning rests my mind."

Cleaning lets us create order out of chaos, which, given how much chaos we encounter every day, feels good.

You don't have to be a perfectionist about it. Maximize your cleaning impact by choosing one room. Put on some music and clear out the errant toys, the dated magazines, the empty cups. Thrill to find that overdue library book or that bag of cosmetics you'd forgotten you bought. When the room is clean—good-enough clean, not perfect—take a moment to breathe it in.

See If Affirmations Will Work for You

Our thoughts are powerful influences on how we feel, how we see the world, how we see ourselves. Thoughts can't make a rainy day sunny, but they can help us be sunny under the umbrella.

Many things—our conditioning, our personalities, how others interact with us, illnesses, beliefs—affect our thoughts. Affirmations are intentional phrases that affirm a reality or viewpoint we want to nurture.

Maybe you've tried affirmations before, believing (as they're often touted) that affirmations are the answer for all ills if you do them "perfectly." Maybe they made you cheerful for a little while, and then life went back to normal. Maybe you tried them once, but they seemed forced.

There isn't a "perfect" way to do affirmations. Try different phrasings to make them work for you. For instance, when you're tired, try saying "I feel energized and alive throughout my body." Does that change the level of energy or does it bring up the contrary view? Maybe it will work better to honor the process, not the outcome: "I am becoming more energized each day."

For some, writing affirmations makes them bright in their mind. For others, speaking them aloud or into a tape player makes them resonate. Find the best way for you.

Tap on Your Collarbone

Western science is beginning to codify how acupuncture works. According to the National Center for Complementary and Alternative Medicine, acupuncture and acupressure conduct electromagnetic signals at points on the body to activate innate pain-relief systems and change the release of neurotransmitters and hormones whereby a person's blood pressure, blood flow, and body temperature are regulated.

You can touch, massage, tap, or even thump your own acupressure points to reenergize yourself, help you focus, and increase your vitality. The place to start, according to energy practitioner Donna Eden, are points on the kidney meridian. The points are located just below the prominences of the inner clavicle (collar bone). Don't worry about getting the exact spot. Tap or massage these indents with the fingertips. (Use fingers of opposite hands if you'd like, or your thumb and fingers if you have only one hand free.)

You can boost the effect, says Eden, by pulling upward on these points with one hand while simultaneously pulling up slightly on your naval with the middle finger of your other hand. You don't even have to understand why it works to enjoy it.

Weed

Weeding is more than making your garden look nice for passersby. And it's more than taming the spread of errant plants. The process of weeding clears your mind, gives you space—in the guise of giving your plants space—to take hold and deepen roots, to support what's really important and cull out the rest.

You can weed away fatigue, critical thoughts, blocks, and annoyances as you pull dandelions, chickweed, and clover. Weeding helps you breathe. You literally touch the earth, feeling part of the energy of growth. Maybe that's why God invented weeds.

Watch Your Caffeine Intake

Face it: Caffeine works. It increases alertness, reduces sensations of fatigue and boredom, and allows you to continue longer with repetitive or exhausting tasks. It pumps you up. But at a price. It also dilates your blood vessels, increases your heart and respiratory rate, and produces more stomach acid. Higher doses have been shown to cause nervousness, anxiety, disturbed sleep, and ulcers, and it may aggravate PMS in women.

Caffeine reliance usually brings an inevitable letdown. For many morning coffee drinkers, the letdown comes in mid afternoon. But afternoon caffeine can affect your night's sleep—a catch 22.

You don't have to quit caffeine totally. Instead, gradually eliminate one serving of coffee or one cola per day, until you are getting no more than 300 milligrams of caffeine. Experiment with substitutes. If you're a coffee drinker, try black or green tea or ginseng tea. If cola's your caffeine of choice, try a different soda. Make half-decaf and half-regular drinks as a transition. As you moderate your reliance on ingested stimulants, you might find hidden energy reserves. Meanwhile, do at least one energy booster that you know works for you. And try out new ones each day to increase your repertoire.

Bend Forward

The seated forward bend yoga pose, according to *Yoga Journal*, can "help a distracted mind unwind" as well as soothe headaches, anxiety, and reduce fatigue, among other benefits. It's a simple pose to describe: You sit on the floor, legs out, and reach for your toes. But it should be done mindfully to get the most benefit and least strain—and not done at all if you have lower back problems.

Start by sitting on the floor, your sit bones raised slightly on a small pillow, folded towel, or blanket. Press into the floor with your hip bones; extend into the sky with your spine and the crown of your head. Press outward through your heels. Already you should feel an energizing stretch.

Hug your thigh muscles to your bones. Inhale as you raise your arms up over your head. Exhale, bend the knees slightly, and from your pelvis, reach toward the toes, ankles, or shins (or a belt or strap around your feet, if that's more comfortable). Don't collapse your chest, keep your heart open. Hold for three to six breaths, feeling a slight stretch in your legs. If you'd like, bend the knees enough to support your head, and then hold for another three to six breaths. When you're ready, uncurl your spine, feeling the pelvis sink into the earth, letting the head come up last. Feel unwound?

Play a Game

Want more energy? Find a kid. Play with one! Kids' play, like improvisational theater, makes life a game to enjoy, not a task to complete. As Shakespeare said, "All the world's a stage, and all the [boys and girls] merely players."

A familiar game—basketball, swings, Legos—can turn into something unexpected. Basketball becomes the knight's jousting lance. The swing becomes the birds' wings. The Lego boat becomes the magical vehicle going into the center of the earth.

Let your own childlike self join in. Match the child's pace and ideas, then begin to add new twists. Just as in improv theater, eliminate the tendency to say "no," with "yes, and . . ." Yes, the basketball wins the joust, and that gives you a magical new sword! And me one too! If you can't connect with children you know, go sit near a sandbox. Marvel at how the toy trucks fly or dig deep into the dark earth! It's a step outside that zings your normal life.

Rule Out Sleep Apnea

Are you a big snorer? You could be suffering from sleep apnea, a very common and serious disorder in which you actually stop breathing hundreds of times per night. One of the side effects is tiredness because you are not getting restorative sleep. Apnea affects at least eighteen million Americans, both men and women, according to the National Sleep Foundation, and is most commonly treated by surgery.

How do you know if you have it? It is usually accompanied by very loud snoring. See *www.sleepfoundation.org*. If you suspect you have it, get thee to a doctor, pronto.

Open Your Shoulders

Opening up the shoulders and chest is a good way to get oxygen and circulation going to enliven the body and spirit. This stretch is great when you're fatigued from a day sitting or hunched over a book.

    Stand if you can, or try this on a stool or low-backed chair. Interlace your fingers behind your back, palms facing in and tight toward each other. Straighten your arms out behind you as you raise them. Make sure you stand tall (don't lean forward) and keep your lower back long—tuck your pelvis up. Don't push yourself beyond a range that feels like a good stretch. Squeeze your shoulder blades together and open up your chest. Take three to five breaths. Relax, then repeat one or more times.

Don't Hit the Snooze Button!

It's better to set the alarm for the time you really want to get up, rather than waking up and going back to sleep for a few minutes. Why? Because your body has just the right amount of time to go into the deepest sleep before being yanked out of it by the buzzer again. Then you end up feeling groggier than you would have if you'd just gotten up the first time.

Make Sure You're Not
Clinically Depressed

One of the common symptoms of depression is fatigue. If you have no reason to feel draggy all the time and have tried many things to no avail, perhaps you should rule out depression. There are many mood drugs now available so you don't have to suffer. And it doesn't mean you have to be on drugs forever. Dr. Bonnie Strickland, past president of the American Psychological Association, was recently quoted in *Health* magazine saying that "properly treated, two-thirds of folks recover within three or four months."

According to the National Institute of Mental Health, signs of depression include: sadness, hopelessness, and pessimistic or empty feelings; trouble concentrating, making decisions, or remembering; decreased energy and fatigue; inability to sleep or oversleeping; loss of interest in activities you once enjoyed, including sex; significant weight loss or gain; restlessness, irritability, or excessive crying; feelings of helplessness, worthlessness, or guilt; thoughts of death or suicide or suicide attempts; and aches and pains and other physical symptoms that don't respond to treatment.

Eat a Sweet Potato

Research suggests that eating a sweet potato can give you steady energy for up to three hours and cut down your energy sags by half. That's because sweet potatoes have 50 percent more fiber than white potatoes and the fiber slows absorption and allows blood sugar to stay even. Try one for breakfast or lunch and notice the effect.

Do a Right-Angle Bend

Yoga bends refresh and give a burst of energy by bringing blood flow to the head. They also relax and lengthen the back muscles. This right-angle bend uses a chair or desk to support you and deepen the relaxation. Be mindful of back problems—go slowly and accept your own limits.

Take one or two steps away from your desk or a chair that's facing away from you. Stand tall and feel your feet press into the floor. Keeping your chest open and back long, fold at the hips until your hands reach the edge of the desk or the back of the chair. Let your shoulder blades slide down your back. Take four to six long, smooth breaths.

When you're ready, step forward into a standing position. You should feel the surge of blood and energy in your arms, chest, and legs.

Cut Down on Copper

Yes, most of our diets contain copper and too much can cause tiredness. Copper is found in foods that otherwise are great— shellfish, soy products, and tea. So if you are trying to eat right and have increased your consumption of any of these, try backing off of them a bit and see if you have more energy.

Collapse

Some days, you just feel like collapsing. And some days it makes sense to follow that urge, then catch the updraft of renewal. Here's a good way to collapse and stretch, even in a private moment at work.

Sit on the front of your chair and position your legs so they are wider than hip-distance apart. Sit up tall, then bend forward from the hip crease keeping your back long. When your lower back is as far forward as it will go (without falling off the chair) let your hands, shoulders, and head relax toward the floor. Your back will round as you drop your head and completely relax your neck. You may have your palms on the floor or on your calves. If there's a pinching or discomfort between your thighs and stomach, place a rolled-up towel or small blanket at the crease of the hip and try again.

Let the tension drain toward the floor with each exhalation, relaxing your body and mind more and more. When you're ready to come back upright, do it slowly as you inhale. (If you need more than one inhale to become fully upright, pause as you exhale and move during the next inhale.) Feel the impetus come from your pelvis, keeping your neck and head dropped until you are fully upright.

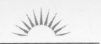

Try TAT

When we're stuck in a loop of panic or mental arguments or depression, it can drain every other aspect of our lives. We might know intellectually that we have to feel the feelings and let them go, but when we try, the feelings don't let go. They intensify or spiral. A simple and elegant technique, originated by acupuncturist Tapas Fleming, allows you to feel safe to release the disturbing emotions and sensations. More information about TAT (Tapas Acupressure Techniques) is available at *www.tat-intl.com* or in Fleming's book *You Can Heal Now*.

Simply place the thumb and ring finger of one hand on either side of the bridge of your nose, and rest your middle finger in the center of your forehead. With your other hand, hold the base of your skull—the occipital ridge. You can do this lying, standing, or sitting, and you can switch hands as needed.

Now intensify the sensation that's been disturbing you. Focus on the physical sensation, image, or dialogue that captures the discomfort. Keep coming back to the disturbance and intensifying it until you find that it has lessened its hold. It might take a minute, it might take twenty. Then remove your hands, take a breath, and see if the intensity has lessened or your relationship to the discomfort has changed. If not, do another round or two of TAT to see if it helps. When the feelings let go, you will feel lighter and more able to move ahead with your life.

Say Hello to Your Natural Self

Connecting with nature isn't just a luxury—it helps you heal faster and have less stress so you can really do what you want. It's a hard-wired brain connection called biophilia—an affinity with plants, animals, and landscapes.

Researchers have found that watching an aquarium—or even a still hedge—can bring about lower blood pressure or higher brain relaxation. Even a view of the outside world can cause shorter hospital stays. Which is why those corner offices are sought after.

Get a nature energy boost in small or grand ways. Go outside, have lunch by some greenery, get a goldfish, take a hike in a park or wilderness area, put a landscape up on your cubicle wall. Tap into the innate power of nature.

Remember a Peak Experience

What nourishes you? What puts the bubbles in your beer? And how can you get more of it? Tap into what lights you up by recalling a peak experience. An experience where you were delighted to be alive. What was happening at that time? What were you doing, who was with you? Most important, what was your experience like—what you saw, heard, felt.

Simply tapping into and remembering a peak experience can put the zing back in your day. But take it a step further. What else can you do this week to have some of that feeling again? If you were on a boat, maybe a swim will give you some water feeling. If you were in love, maybe you can do a random act of kindness. If you were relaxed on a vacation, maybe you can meditate, or visit an unexplored corner of town or a new park.

Let your peak experience be your guide to gathering up more of what makes you outrageously joyful.

Rotate Your Hips

Sitting at a desk for hours is hard on the body. With a small range of motion, our spines compress and we end up slumping. Even the most petite feel pressure in the buttocks and hips. It can feel as if all the energy gets stuck there.

Simple isometric exercises—contracting and holding the buttock muscles for four to six breaths—livens the area up. But even better are hip rolls. Stand with feet a bit wider than your hips. Circle your pelvis five times one way, then five another. If you're comfortable, do five more each way really wide, feeling the stretch in your hamstrings and legs as you rotate. Do a few figure eights in each direction. And finish off with a little shimmy. Or get a hula hoop! You'll feel like a new person when you sit down again.

Tap into the Vision Thing

What's your vision for your life? Not your plans laid out like stepping stones. Not a goal for a house, career, and 2.3 kids. A vision does not live in the intellect only. Vision is deeper than that. You might know you have a vision for your life, you may have one and not know it, or you may still be developing one. Knowing your vision or the possibility of its existence vitalizes your days beyond any number of grande lattes. It gives your life a sense of motion and purpose.

To get more in touch with it, ask creative questions. Like: If your vision was music, what would it be? If your vision was from nature, would it be a tree, a brook, the ocean . . . ? If your vision was a food, how would it taste? How would a six-year-old describe your vision? What's the wackiest thing about your vision? How will it feel to be truly in your vision? What's one thing you've already done toward your vision? And one thing you can do this week to really make your vision part of your life? That vision thing can be pretty exciting.

Thump Your Thymus

The thymus gland, located above the heart, is central to the functioning of the immune system. Research has theorized that the thymus gland functions to activate white blood cells, T cells, which in turn promote immunity.

ENERGY
BOOSTER

218

People under stress often put a hand over this area. Some energy practitioners encourage tapping the thymus gland to stimulate energy, boost the immune system, and increase vitality.

Your thymus lies under your sternum, a few inches down from your collarbone. Tap this area using four fingers, then use the other hand if desired for a total of about twenty seconds.

Tarzan power without the vines?

Tell Yourself You Feel Great

Believe it or not, the more you say you are tired, the more physically fatigued you will feel. That's because our body/mind/spirit are not separate; we just think they are. If you tell yourself you feel energized, you will give yourself an instantaneous boost.

Try a Banana

Franca Alphin, a clinical dietitian at Duke University, touts bananas as a great energy booster. That's why tennis players eat them so often between sets. The lift comes from fruit sugar, and the effect lasts up to two hours. Best of all, for us folks always on the go, they're super easy to carry. And they're great for an afternoon snack for kids.

The Old Eight Glasses Advice

The reason so many of us feel tired? We're dehydrated. And what is the relationship between drinking water and feeling energized? The more water in your system, the more oxygen circulates in your bloodstream. So be sure to drink those eight glasses of water you've been hearing about for years. (And no, coffee and soda don't count.)

Stretch Your Armpits

Want to know the oddest place we hold tension? The armpits. When we open and stretch this area, we open the chest, stimulate the lymph glands, and just feel better.

Here's a stretch you probably naturally gravitate toward. It's a full-body stretch when done standing (feet shoulder-width apart). But it also works in a chair.

Raise your arms toward the ceiling as you inhale. Interlace your fingers, and then roll your palms outward. Relax your shoulders and breathe. Now inhale and stretch toward your left—relax those shoulders! After a few breaths, return to center on an inhale and repeat the stretch to your right. Come back to center.

As you exhale, lower your arms down and feel the relaxation and openness in your body.

ENERGY
BOOSTER

222

You Need Vitamin D

According to the Vitamin D Skin and Bone Research Lab at Boston Medical Center, we need up to 1,000 IU a day of vitamin D, which is much more than the federally recommended dose of 200–400 IU. And that vitamin D deficiency can lead to feeling depleted, achy bones, depression, and even chronic fatigue and fibromyalgia.

Because 90 percent of our body's supply of vitamin D comes from ultraviolet rays through skin, it is crucial that we go out in the sun for five to ten minutes (ten to twenty for dark skin) without sunscreen between eleven a.m. and two p.m. at least two to three times a week (and every day during the winter when the sun is weak). More than that and we're at increased risk for skin cancer. But less than that, we're not getting the vitamin D we need. If you're not sure if you are getting enough, you can take a supplement. But be sure to take it with food to get maximum absorption.

Sniff an Orange

Really. When your mental energy is flagging and you must keep on concentrating, sniffing certain smells actually can increase attention. So says the Smell and Taste Treatment and Research Foundation. Try citrus—an orange, lemon, lime, or grapefruit half. Fresh rosemary, jasmine, ginger, eucalyptus, spearmint, or peppermint also work.

Become Your Own Coach

If you stepped into a magical hot-air balloon that let you see your life from a high perspective, what would you notice that you miss day to day?

Unless we have a personal life coach or therapist or outrageous friend, we don't often step out to see ourselves in new ways. To see what drains or clouds our energy. To see what vitalizes us. But you can be your own outrageous friend and ask yourself some outrageous questions and get a new enlivening perspective.

Try questions like these from the Coaches Training Institute: Who inspires you and why? What would your life be like if you had unlimited time and resources? What needs in the world would you like to serve? What makes you feel powerful? When do you give your power away? What drives you crazy? What delights you?

Let the questions create sparks that can illuminate where you want to go next.

Let There Be Light

Studies have shown that if you put your bedside light on a timer to turn on about one hour before you wake up, you'll wake up more energized. So give it a try and see how you feel!

Get Computer Glasses

If you spend most of the day looking at the computer screen—as more and more of us do—you may notice eye strain (blurred vision, double vision, stinging eyes), headaches, or neck and shoulder pain. All of these can zap our ability to be productive and creative. Some of this can be corrected with a glare screen or changing the resolution of the monitor. But computer glasses can really take the fatigue out of working.

Computer glasses help your eyes focus restfully on the monitor's midrange between close reading work and the distance vision you use when driving. Some computer glasses function as bifocals or trifocals: the bottom for reading, the mid level for computer, and the top for distance, so you can wear them for all your tasks. Even if you don't yet need glasses for vision or reading, computer glasses can help prevent eye burnout.

Yes, Exercise

Unless you've been living under a rock, this energy booster will not be new information. Instead think of it as a reminder, an encouragement, an inducement to do what you already know your body needs for energy: exercise.

Here's inducement for your brain: Fitness improves cognition and concentration. For your emotions: Exercise improves your mood, reduces depression and anxiety, relieves stress, increases endorphins, decreases tension, and helps you sleep. For your appearance: It increases muscle mass, reduces fat, increases range of motion, makes your skin glow, helps you appear more vibrant. For your body in general: Exercise increases your energy level and stamina, helps you resist fatigue and disease, and increases your metabolism.

What, how, and when? Start small and easy—walking ten minutes a day, a drop-in beginner's aerobics or yoga class, dancing in your living room. Do it regularly, at least three or four times a week so your body remembers how great it feels to move. Scan the Internet or the community-center calendar to explore new exercise options: rowing, in-line skating, NIA (freestyle meditative dance), deep water aerobics. Take walks with friends instead of meeting at a coffee shop. Put stickers on your calendars when you exercise so you can see the reality of your commitment. Don't do it perfectly, don't think about it—just do it. You'll feel the upsurge in energy.

Stop

"Let's go. C'mon. Hurry up." How many times have you said that to your kids, drivers on the road, yourself? It's not just our culture and to-do lists that keep us jumping from one task to another or several at once. It's our own drive and discomfort—or unfamiliarity—with who we are when we stop.

When your energy is low—or when it's not—just stop. Where are you? How are you feeling? What are you thinking? What's real and what do you imagine?

One man said, "Stopping is the hardest thing to do, to just be present and accept who I am, where I am and when I am." But that acceptance is the power behind moving forward.

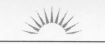

Cool Your Jets

Heat can be enervating, making people languish like over-cooked linguini (in fact, doctors are discovering that there are folks with reverse Seasonal Affective Disorder; rather than becoming depressed in the winter, the bright light and heat of summer brings them down). Even with refreshing air conditioning, the body must use energy to make constant quick adjustments from a cool seventy degrees to a humid ninety-six. Here are some ways to keep your cool when you can't rely on air conditioners:

1. Stay hydrated: Drink water and iced teas. Eat fruit. Be aware that alcohol and caffeine have dehydrating effects.
2. Keep your curtains closed during the day, open them at night.
3. Lie on a cool floor. Your whole body will release the heat, especially if it's a tile floor—and the change in perspective (remember imagining walking on the ceiling as a kid?) will revitalize you.
4. Eat frozen peas or berries.
5. Before you go to sleep, take a tepid or cool shower. Dab off, then sleep on your damp towel on your bed.
6. Put an ice bag or cool "gel sheets" (designed for migraines) on your forehead, back of your neck, wrists, or behind your knees.

Change the Color of Your Walls

Color subtly enlivens the senses and affects moods. In the science of physics, colors correspond to electromagnetic frequencies of oscillation: red is low frequency, violet high, and yellow in between. From a human perspective, we tend to have associations with different colors—red may evoke passion; pink, innocence; black, seriousness. However, color reactions are highly individual, related to cultural background, gender, and (when working in a colorful room) ability to screen out stimuli.

The most enriching and luminous atmospheres reflect the full spectrum of nature. This doesn't mean a blue ceiling, green carpet, red chairs, and yellow walls—although in certain hues it might. It means bringing in texture, gradations of color, and warm and cool tones.

Changing the color in your living or work space can give you more energy by heightening your positive color reactions. Check out the paint store chips. (If you're overwhelmed by the myriad choices, you might want to find a color consultant.) Before you paint the room, be sure to try a large swatch on the walls to see how the color looks in morning, evening, and artificial light. And remember, you can paint just one wall, like the wall behind your computer monitor, for a splash of liveliness to sail through the day.

You May Have Diabetes

If you have tried all kinds of things and still feel exhausted all the time, perhaps you are one of the six million Americans who have undiagnosed adult-onset diabetes. Diabetes, a disease caused by the body's inability to produce or use insulin, is not something to ignore—it can destroy your kidneys, cause blindness, quadruple your chance of heart attack and stroke, and lead to leg amputations. The American Diabetes Association reports that about seventeen million folks suffer currently from diabetes and estimates that this figure will rise by one million every year.

The reason? Primarily obesity. But even those who aren't obese are at risk—a gain of eleven to eighteen pounds doubles the chance that you will develop type 2 diabetes, the most common form. Doctors are now recommending that everyone be tested for type 2 every three years starting at age forty-five; if you are tired all the time, overweight and inactive, have high blood pressure or a family history of diabetes, or are African American, Native American, or Hispanic (the highest risk ethnic groups), you should be tested earlier and more often. The test is a blood test done after an overnight fast to measure your blood sugar level.

Make Your Own Music

Even if you hated piano lessons as a child, your guitar is collecting dust in the closet, or you've never touched a musical instrument, making music is amazingly empowering. Pull out an old friend like Bach's Minuet in G. Visit a music store for the visual and auditory delights while you check out music books for adult beginners. If you've never played, try banging a drum or twiddle with some easy instruments like an ocarina, recorder, or thumb piano. You don't have to be Yo-Yo Ma, Duke Ellington, or Nora Jones to get the uplift from making music.

Get a Massage

If you don't have time for a full hour massage, get a mini one. Fifteen-minute chair massages loosen your neck and shoulders. You sit in a special massage chair and lean into padded neck and shoulder rests. Loose shoulders release the body's energy. Large corporations, office parks, and airports often offer quick massages. Or you can call a recommended massage therapist and ask.

Tap Your Spleen

According to Chinese medicine, the spleen meridian or energy channel governs the assimilation of nutrients from food and fluids. Tapping or stretching this meridian has been encouraged by Shiatsu and energy practitioners for balancing blood chemistry, strengthening the immune system, removing toxins, and increasing energy.

The spleen points are located below your nipples, about one rib below your breasts; they are likely to be a bit tender. If you use several fingertips together, you'll stimulate the area enough to not be too concerned about the exact spot. You can tap on these points for about fifteen seconds.

Another way to stimulate the spleen meridian is to stretch backward in your chair or on the floor (with your feet under your buttocks and knees together). Clasp your hands, turn the palms out, and raise your arms up high overhead and then stretch them behind you. Breathe and feel the opening in this meridian. When you're done, notice the vitality returning to your central core.

Wrestle

We grapple with a lot each day—deadlines, priorities, sassy kids, the queue at the grocery store. It can be freeing to playfully let our bodies express it.

If you have elementary-school-age children or nieces and nephews, play fight with them. Say "grrrrrr." Try to pin each other down. Be silly. It's important as an adult for you to match their level of strength and keep it physically and emotionally safe. But channeling mild aggression into play is a release that feels great—for both adults and kids.

If you have a partner, wrestling can be a great way to let go of tension accumulated in and out of the relationship. Again, matching levels of strength and keeping it safe.

Maybe a Body Pillow Would Help

A good night's sleep is the foundation for rejuvenation. And for great sleeping comfort, some swear by a body pillow.

A body pillow is a full-length pillow that can go from neck to knees, or even curl in a C shape around your whole body. Use it to prop under your shoulder, your hip, and between your knees to take pressure off stress spots and relieve back pain as you sleep on your side. You can get a similar effect from several individual pillows, but that requires more fuss when you turn over at three in the morning.

First "discovered" by pregnant women, body pillows have become widely available—there are even ones with baseball logos! It's worth it to have a great night's sleep.

Get Your Hands on Some Yarn

There's something energizing about knitting and needlework—feeling the yarn on your fingers, immersing in colors, the routine percussion of needles, the creation of something (which may or may not turn out to be useful), the portability of doing it at meetings or while waiting. There is even a rumor about a medical student who knitted in lectures instead of taking notes—and did better than most of her classmates.

Because of the rhythmic, repetitive stitching and the needles clicking at regular intervals, knitting is a "calming mantra" says Harvard Medical School professor Dr. Herbert Benson in his book *The Relaxation Response*. "Working with yarn provides stress relief."

Knitting and needlework can be solitary or be part of a community. If you've never done it before, join a class at a community center or a yarn shop. Most shops welcome people working on projects to get help and even sit a spell.

If you're an experienced needle-crafter with a closet of half-done products you tell yourself you have to finish, pick up an unfinished project and see if it takes root in your heart as you work it. Or donate your old yarn to a senior center and find a new project to thrill you. Enjoy the process and the product will likely come out better as well. Knit one, purl two, and revitalize.

See Green

A growing body of experiments are showing that looking at the greenery of nature helps children and adults pay attention better and have more energy to deal with problems. You don't even have to be out very long. "We're seeing that amazingly you can detect effects even after not very much exposure," said Frances Kuo of the University of Illinois at Urbana-Champaign. "Even 20 minutes in a somewhat green place seems to be better than those same 20 minutes indoors." No wonder so many folks can't do without their weekly golf game!

Release the Bottleneck

Pent-up anger takes a lot of energy to manage. You have to contain your verbal and body language; you get stiff from keeping it in. We might believe that getting our anger out—storming or confronting the person we think has harmed us—will make us feel better. And in some ways it does, if just momentarily. There is the relief from not holding it in; there is the perverse sense of company from knowing someone else is angry too. But studies show that often this kind of release escalates the problem and the anger.

Some people think anger is bad and try to avoid thinking about it. But anger is a natural, adaptive response to threats, and a certain amount of it is wired in to our survival. One way to experience and release our anger without involving anyone else is to move and notice our bodies.

Anger is held in the pelvis, hands, and jaw according to Dr. Alexander Lowen, a founder of the field of Bioenergetics. He suggests lying on your back, pounding your fists and hips into the bed. Or take a brisk walk, swinging your fists and saying aloud or to yourself, "No. No. No!" Or notice anger in your body when swimming, kneading bread dough (one less appliance), or even doing yoga. Let yourself feel your anger without explaining or arguing against it. Notice the sensations as they arise and ebb. Afterward, you may be able to reclaim your energy and take calm action, if you still need to.

Give the Dog the Boot

Studies have shown that folks who sleep with their pets have more trouble sleeping than others because they keep getting woken up. (We bet the same is true for parents of little children!) Find another place for Fido to bed down for the night. (By the way, dog trainers will tell you that you will have a more obedient dog if you kick him out of the bed; otherwise, he thinks you're all pack equals. This way, he'll know you're in charge.)

Exercise Late in the Day

Whether you run or do other aerobic activity, scientists have found that if you do heavy exercise late in the day, the heat you generate will allow you to fall sleep faster and stay more soundly asleep. That's why heating yourself up with a hot bath also works.

Wake Up Your Body with the Cat-Cow

The name of this basic yoga pose comes from the two alternating positions: a mooing cow (you don't have to moo) and a puffed-up cat with a rounded back. The cat pose has a calming effect, the cow pose more stimulating—and the combination, balancing.

Start on your hands and knees on the floor with your hands directly under your shoulders and knees under your hips. Use a blanket or towel if your knees are tender. All motion in this pose starts with the movement in the pelvis and uses strong abdominal muscles throughout, to prevent swaying your back too much.

Exhale the air from your lungs. Inhale as you do the cow pose: tilt the pelvis forward, press with your hands to open your chest, and let your head look upward in line with your spinal curve. Exhale as you reverse into cat pose: tuck your pelvis—as if you're putting your tail between your legs—so your spine rounds. Press with your hands to open the back of your heart, and allow your head to drop. Let your motions be fluid with a long, smooth breath. Repeat the series six to ten times.

Take Up Yoga

Yoga, the ancient Hindu system of exercises to train both the consciousness and the body, has been practiced for millennia. You can get a lot from just a little yoga. In recent decades, researchers have found that yoga improves attention, memory, endurance, and concentration. It decreases pain, blood pressure, pulse rate, depression, and anxiety. In addition, yoga balances the digestion, improves range of motion, and is both calming and invigorating.

ENERGY
BOOSTER

244

A regular class, weekly or more often, is best for learning the moves and getting individualized feedback on postures and injury prevention. Once you know the poses, practicing at home—on your own or with a book, CD, or video—helps energize you between, or instead of, classes.

There are many styles of yoga: flowing Vinyasa, precise Iyengar, sweat-inducing Bikram, awareness-focused Forrest, power-generating Astanga, heart-filled Anusara, and more. If you have an affinity for yoga in general, most styles will provide benefits of energized calm. But certain styles and teachers will probably increase your enjoyment and progress. Check out friends, the phone book, natural food stores, alternative magazines, and health clubs for a place to start. And gain the wisdom and energy of the 5,000-year-old tradition.

Lower Your Information Overload

Information is a double-edged sword. Enough of it helps you make decisions, too much makes you second-guess yourself. Enough helps you do your job, too much and you're spending all your time filtering it. Enough makes you feel informed to manage your world, too much makes you feel dread and paralysis. Too much information siphons your energy.

Everyone makes individual decisions about how to get their information and what's enough—from those who shut themselves off from the daily flow to those who love swimming in it. Ask yourself: What's important to know and when? Are you drowning in too much information? What's enough for you? If you set some criteria, you won't have to decide if each interaction is worth checking into.

You can list your phone number on the national Do Not Call Registry. You can toss or shred junk mail without opening it. You can get your news from the paper (where you can scan at your own pace, not that of the news director). Your trashcan will get full when you manage your information. But so will your energy.

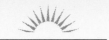

Turn Off That Inner Critic

Sit down, pour a cup of tea, and have a conversation with your critic. Your critic is that inner alarm that rings—or yells or whines—every time you step out of its ever shifting safety zone. Your critic zaps your energy with twisted logic and persistent arguments, inner sabotage, option overload, and constant fear and disapproval.

There are several things that help you rescue your energy from the critic. The first is to notice it. Where do you feel the critic in your body? Is it a voice? Does it have a body? A name? Maybe it's an oozing little warty troll named Grumble that likes to hang out in your stomach and whine complaints and criticisms about all you do or don't do. By noticing your critic, you realize that you exist outside of it—and that is where you get your power to live your life.

Second, talk back. This is not the same as arguing with your critic because, frankly, your critic is a lot better at winning arguments than you are. But just as you would if your child condemned you for not letting her play in traffic, you say, "That's not true. I'm not bad, and I'm not going to justify it to you." Then inform your critic that you are changing the rules. You will listen to it at crucial times, but it's moving to the back seat. You're not getting rid of the critic—that just feeds the battle—but you're reorganizing its place in your life. You're in the driver's seat with the energy for where you really want to go.

Let Your Spine Ooze

Letting your spine "ooze" is a great way to loosen up the vertebrae, get the spinal fluid going, and enliven yourself.

You can do it in a chair with your hands on a table or desk, but start the first time by getting the basic sensation on the floor. Position yourself on your hands and knees, using a towel or blanket if your knees are tender. Keep your hands directly beneath your shoulders and your knees directly below or a little wider than your hips. Start straightening and bending your elbows, rocking side to side or making circles with your chest. Let the movements grow larger so you rock back toward your feet or forward toward your hands. Use your abdominal muscles to keep the back stable. Remember to breathe and to keep your neck and shoulders relaxed (dropping down your back). You should feel stretches in your legs, arms, spine, and torso as you do this.

As you're ready to stop, make the movements smaller. Come back to hands and knees and notice how you feel. Rise up slowly, with awareness of your fluid, enlivened spine.

Fire Up with a Fruit Smoothie

In her book *Natural Energy*, Dr. Erika Schwartz offers the following recipe for a breakfast drink that will keep your brain alert:

4 oz. water
4 oz. orange juice
1 scoop whey protein
1 cup frozen mixed berries
1 banana
a few ice cubes

Combine all in a blender and mix until smooth.

Soak Your Feet

Remember the feeling of wading into a cold stream on a hot sunny day? Your toes tingle, your feet pulse, your whole body glows. When the weather is warm, you can get that feeling even without trekking to a brook. Fans of hydrotherapy (one of the oldest and simplest tonics) suggest a cold foot soak—or even better, alternating hot and cold soaks—to reduce swelling and enliven the feet and legs as well as stimulate the entire circulatory system. Hydrotherapy is said to increase lymph circulation, tone body tissues, relax the nerves, and improve health. And a foot soak feels great.

You can bring a basin of cold water to wake up tired tootsies while watching television—or sit on the edge of the bath with your feet in a few inches of cold water. Or try it hot: soak in comfortably hot water for five to twenty minutes—adding hot water as needed to maintain the temperature. Finish off by rinsing your feet under a cold tap.

And you don't even need to stub your toe falling off a slippery rock.

Scrub with Salt

Pampering yourself, moisturizing your body, stimulating your skin, exfoliating dead cells, emanating a glow—quite a charge from a little rub with a bit of salt and maybe oil.

Salt scrubs have taken on new cachet, touted as hot treatments at the best spas. You can buy salt scrubs at health and cosmetic stores. And you can concoct your own salt scrub to see how invigorating it can be after a shower or bath.

Start with a handful of kosher table salt, or Epsom salts (or a mixture) in a bowl. The larger the salt grains, the rougher the scrub. Add a tablespoon or two of oil. Almond is often suggested, but in a "what's-handy" experiment, try canola or olive. A fragrant oil, like peppermint, adds sensual stimulation. Let the mixture sit for a few hours, until it's moist with just a little oil floating on top. (If it's too greasy or dry, you can always add more salt or oil.)

After your bath or shower, rub the mixture into your damp skin. Begin at the feet and work up, avoiding scratched or wounded areas. ("Salt in the wounds" is not an adage for nothing.) Massage your legs, stomach, chest, arms, neck, and lightly on your face. Then rinse with warm or cool water and towel off.

Enjoy your delicious self-marinade.

It Could Be the Pill Is to Blame

Women: birth control pills can cause a buildup of minerals in your bloodstream, which can block your body's absorption of essential nutrients, thus making you tired. How can you find out if that's going on? One way is through a hair analysis, in which a strand of hair is analyzed to see what elements are present. This test is controversial, however, with many mainstream physicians pooh-poohing its diagnostic relevance.

Revive Mentally with a Toy

What products are designed expressly to stimulate your thinking, engage your imagination, heighten your visual acuity, make you smile—and can cost as little as a quarter? Toys!

Wander through a toy store and see what's new and what brings back memories, from pot holder looms to an electronic stapler kit. Buy some Legos to build a beach cruiser or a scene from your wedding. Get a new yo-yo. Or a mini fire extinguisher at Office Playground ("fun stuff for your desk"). Check out the Ben Franklin action figure—with a key and kite—at Archie McPhee's fabulous Web site (*www.mcphee.com*) for zany adults and kids.

Toys are designed to make kids say, "I want to play with that!" And they have the same effect on adults. Let the smile on your face and the creative break offer you room to play with your life.

ENERGY
BOOSTER

252

Cuddle

Wake up your nerve endings by cuddling with a partner, child, dog, or cat. Being physically close to loved ones can connect you to positive body sensations and to the affection in the world around you.

Pack a Snack

Carry healthy snacks in your purse or briefcase, so you can eat
something at the first sign of afternoon tiredness. Hardboiled
eggs, low-fat protein bars, dried fruit, and beef and turkey
jerky are all good choices. This will also help you stay away
from high-fat snacks that are bad for your waistline as well as
your energy levels.

Water Yourself

Keep a spray bottle of water in your desk or car. A spritz on your arms and/or face will instantly revive you.

Get Enough Niacin

When you can't make use of your body's fuel, you're like a car with clogged spark plugs trying to accelerate on the freeway. No matter how hard you push the pedal to the floor you get jolts and hesitations, not smooth sailing. Feel familiar?

A proven essential ingredient to make use of your fuel—food—is vitamin B3, niacin. Niacin helps release the energy from protein, fat, and carbohydrates. It's needed to metabolize some drugs and toxins, as well as to form red blood cells and some hormones. If that weren't enough, niacin also promotes the health of the digestive tract, central nervous system, and skin.

So eat your protein (lean beef, fish, poultry), dairy products, B3-enriched bread and cereals, nuts, and eggs. Try some brewers yeast on your stir-fry.

Or take a supplement that includes the recommended dose for adults of fourteen to sixteen milligrams per day of niacin.

Make a U-Turn

A simple yoga inversion—a yoga pose where you put your heart above your head—stretches your spine, brings blood flow to the brain, and gives you a new perspective. Like making your body do a U-turn. Stand with your feet hip-width apart, pointed forward. Inhale. On the exhale, slowly drop your head, and then continue to curl your spine down until you're hanging over. (Bend your knees slightly if your hamstrings behind your thighs feel too tight.) Place your hands on your thighs, your calves, the floor, or even grab your big toe if you're limber enough. Or spread your feet wider than hip-width and rest your palms on the floor.

Another option is to put your hands on a chair you've placed in front of you. (You can rest your head on the chair or a cushion for extra restorative time.) Relax your neck so your head hangs. Take three to ten breaths, feeling your body stretching and opening. Play with where the weight is on your feet—your balls or your heels, the inside or outside—to change the stretch. When you're ready to rise, exhale first. Then as you inhale, uncurl, starting at your pelvis (keeping your head hanging). If you run out of breath before you're all the way up, pause and exhale before you continue on a new inhalation. When you're standing, take a breath or two and feel your energy.

Hire an Organizer

Pampering yourself with a massage, facial, even an extra professional housecleaning is a great energy boost. But the effects may wane soon after you schlep in the groceries or cook spaghetti sauce. An indulgence with lingering effects—for days, months, or years after—comes from hiring a professional organizer. A professional organizer is not a mob hit man or a political activist. It's a person who helps make decisions and sets up systems in the areas that tend toward chaos—papers, finances, sewing supplies, holiday decorations, linens, basements, pantries.

The short-term energy boost is seeing your file folders in alphabetical order and your desk clear of piled papers. The long-term boost comes months later when you locate your son's vaccination record within minutes.

To find a professional organizer, check the Internet, perhaps the National Association of Professional Organizers (*www.napo.net*). Since you and the organizer will have a rather intimate relationship—after all, you're sharing your hidden, disorganized self—check out potential organizers on the phone for their values, judgments, sense of humor, references. Then get set to experience a more organized life.

Massage Those Digits

Wringing your hands is actually a skill—not just something to do when you're worried. Giving yourself a simple hand massage can enliven your whole body. Shiatsu (Japanese manipulative therapy), reflexology, and other healing disciplines identify energy lines (meridians) that network throughout the body and have reflex points on the hands. Try a hand massage anytime, but especially in the bath or as a break from washing dishes.

Lay the massaging hand across the back of the receiving hand—both hands pointing down, fingers of one hand touching the wrist of the other. With your fingertips, massage between the bones on the back of your hand. Massage the palm with the ball of the thumb, then press hard into the palm with the second knuckles of the index and middle fingers. Now the fingers: Pull and twist each one. Then pinch and rub circles from the fingertip to the base. Grip your wrist and massage it between the fingers and the base of your palm. When you've done both sides, open your hands by pressing your fingertips together, opening wide.

Pay Attention to Pain

Pain saps your energy—it's designed to do that. It's a signal for your body to pay attention, to protect and nurture and heal a part of your body. Pain hits you on all levels: physical sensation, thoughts, emotions, motivation. It can slow activities, increase worries and hopelessness, make you stop. When pain strikes, there is always one thing you can do. It's what your body wants you to do: pay attention.

Paying attention to pain is a paradox, since sometimes it feels as if you can't get away from it. But it can be a healing paradox, giving you a sense of yourself beyond the tension surrounding the pain.

Breathe and get comfortable. Notice where your pain is strongest. Notice if you can sense an image, sound, or movement from the pain. Perhaps you sense a vibration (fast and intense or slow and long). Maybe some words or colors. Or an image like a fire hose or a tight corset. Does the pain come in waves or does it seem more constant?

Notice what thoughts or emotions accompany or trigger the pain. Perhaps you can feel the pain without those thoughts. (For instance, what does pain feel like without worrying, "Is this serious?") When you pay attention, you realize the parts of you that exist beyond the pain, and you gain resources for your healing and energy.

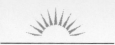

Relax Your Jaw

Some of your strongest muscles are all in your head—your jaw to be precise. The masseter, the temporalis, and the medial pterygoid muscles allowed human forebears to bite, crush, and grind tough, raw food. Now you might be chewing puff pastries or power bars, but those strong muscles may clench when you're awake or asleep. Grinding your boss, perhaps?

This clenching creates tension, worn or fractured teeth, TMJ (temporomandibular joint) disorder, and energy-draining headaches—jaw-clenching muscles in migraine sufferers are 70 percent larger than in others. If you have TMJ (clicking and sticking when you move your jaw), check with your dentist about a tooth guard to wear at night.

When you release your jaw, you unleash your breath, flow of blood and cerebrospinal fluid, and the connection between your head and your body. A simple releasing practice is to remember the words, "Lips together, teeth apart." Let your tongue rest lightly against your front teeth. This position also relaxes tension in the neck and shoulders. Another technique is to soften every facial muscle until your face sags like a basset hound! Try it when you're driving or falling asleep, when no one's looking.

To loosen the jaw, smile broadly then pucker your lips several times. Stick out your tongue, wiggle it side to side then up and down. If you don't have TMJ, jut the jaw out and move it smoothly side to side.

Try a Cold Rub

A cold rub—a hydrotherapy technique that combines cold water, friction, and exfoliation—increases circulation and wakes nerve endings up all over your body. It's also alleged to fortify the immune system. Sounds a little chilling and odd at first but it feels great.

After a hot bath, sauna, or shower, dip a washcloth or small towel in cold water. Wrap the cloth around your hand and rub your other arm in vigorous circles, from the fingers to the shoulder. Your skin will become flushed. You can dry with a fresh towel using the same circular motion, but if you're warm enough, don't bother. Just dip the washcloth in cold water once more and rub the other arm. Then repeat on your feet and legs (toes to thighs), stomach, buttocks, chest, neck, and face (be more gentle here).

If you really like it, you might buy a bath mitt or natural sea sponge to make it a daily invigorating routine.

Declutter Your Finances

Does tax time drain your energy? Unfiled taxes create drag, and not just from the money owed or figuring out what refund is due, or even filling out the 1040.

The stress of taxes often comes from general financial clutter—a box of receipts, an unbalanced checkbook, missing pay stubs, W-2 forms in the glove compartment—you hope. On top of all that might be unexplored feelings about money (especially shame, fear, or anger).

You'll have more energy and feel more hopeful about your money if you use this season to clear up some clutter and your feelings about money. For clutter, you might set up a file for current and next year's taxes. For emotional insight, notice what you think and feel about money as you gather your financial data together. If you can consider new and more nurturing ways to relate to money as you do your taxes, it will be time well invested.

Do You Hear What I Hear?

The buzz of thoughts can supersede just about everything else. As you spin your wheels on inner concepts, you can miss connecting with what's actually in the world. If you take a moment to put your thoughts in the background and just listen, you become more aware of physical reality, feel more relaxed and powerful. Listening opens up all your senses, your creativity, your place in the world.

ENERGY BOOSTER

264

Put your attention on your ears themselves. Notice the sounds around you. Car tires, cell phones, subway trains, footsteps . . . leaves rustling, papers rustling, computer hums, people typing, people talking . . . news shows, reality shows, talk shows, golden oldies, a Mozart sonata . . . water boiling, children playing, robins warbling, lawn mowers, someone whistling. . . .

Close your eyes and notice the three-dimensionality of sound: sounds above and below, left and right, distant and near, faint and loud. Now pay attention to the quietest moments. The silence holding the sound. It's there even in busy places. Noticing silences opens up the mind to the space all around us.

Arrive Early

Rushing can feel like a necessity, not a choice on busy days. Or maybe it's part of your everyday life. Before you leave for an appointment, you just check a few more e-mails, water a plant, complete a spreadsheet—efficient and energy-boosting accomplishments. Or they can create a domino effect of frenzy in your day.

As a change, arrive three to five minutes early for something today. Use the time to gather yourself, relax, make or review notes.

Those occasional minutes can reduce the pace of the whole day. Rather than spending time chasing after missed or almost-missed connections, arriving early lets you have your whole self present for the action at hand—and maybe for more of your day.

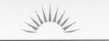

Create a Going-to-Bed Ritual

Insufficient sleep means that you overrely on your adrenaline, your mind, your willpower, and your caffeine to keep going during the day. In charged lives, we want to race around from work to supper to activities, to homework, to TV. Then—hurry up, it's getting late!—brush teeth, iron a shirt, shut off the light, and off to sleep. Except you're still awake.

Sleep and rest require that we slow our movements, increase the hormone melatonin, and move from thinking to processing. But that doesn't automatically happen when we go to bed as if we're turning off the computer. We need to tell our unconscious mind to make that happen. And ritual helps.

What is your going-to-bed ritual? Lowering the lights increases the production of melatonin. Checking the locks, grinding the coffee, brushing your teeth, taking nightly vitamins, soothing the moisturizer on your skin—they all tell your body to start relaxing. Even reading in a lamp-lit room helps letting go. Notice how long it takes you after you start to bed to actually get there. Then several nights this week, begin your nightly ritual early enough to turn lights out for a good night's sleep. Honor the night. It honors you.

Make Faces

Kids do it all the time—despite parents joking that a snooty face will freeze. They make faces when pretending to be knights, are about to get a shot, or get served anchovy sauce or a vanilla ice-cream sundae! They scowl or roll their eyes up or spread their lips out wider than you could imagine. Grown-ups make faces, too, although it can become a frozen habit. Lips pursed waiting for the light to change, eyebrows wrinkled while opening the mail, a pasted grin when the son finally empties the dishwasher. Our faces highlight the information we take in, our emotional reactions, our expectations, and our ability to have flexible responses.

We all have habits, and it's freeing to shake them up. At a stoplight, flex your cheeks, wiggle your lips, raise your eyebrows. Mad at your kid for not listening again? Create a funny, angry face. Amused by the purple crocus flowers? Beam a full-fledged grin from ear to ear. Wish the car ahead would move? Purse your lips out to the end of your nose. Even pretending to have a childlike face of rage, fear, or sadness will loosen your muscles and your emotions. A face and emotions that move means you can quickly respond to what life offers.

Pray

Medical brain scans have shown how we think, feel, prepare, learn—and pray. A part of the human brain gets stimulated when we connect with a sense of the universe beyond the everyday world.

Some think of joy as an undependable gift, bestowed as a raise or a new house or a lover. Others experience a deeper joy by taking time to strengthen their connection to the universe. It doesn't prevent feeling sad, mad, or blue, but it gives the human life a bigger context, a larger play—not just the script of your life's role.

One way to strengthen that connection is through prayer, in its many forms—physical prayer: movement in nature, a Celtic labyrinth puzzle, a religious service, or walking meditation (awareness of each part of the walk, from lifting up the leg to putting it down); visual prayer: imagining a life force, such as God, an angel, or Jesus with you; and the prayer of talking, through conversation or written word, with an image of the force of life. Express gratitude, complain some, ask for help, and tap into a powerful, universal energy that can spark your own vitality.

Juggle

Juggling is not just for kids, clowns, and computer programmers anymore. It actually increases your brain size.

Learning to juggle (try your toy store for books and starter balls) requires focus on rhythm, body, and movement. It feels magical when it works—even just for a few throws. And it takes you away from worrisome thoughts that drain energy.

German scientists researched the brains of people who learned to toss balls in rhythm. Three months after the study, they had a 3 percent increase in the mid-temporal part of the brain (although it decreased by 1 percent once they stopped juggling).

Do the neurons in the brain expand as they form new neural pathways? Does a bigger brain make you smarter? That's still under study. Meanwhile, just throw those three balls around, and know that something's getting better—your motor skills, perception of spatial objects, and fun!

No Naps after Lunch

The urge for a mid-afternoon sleep strikes some strongly. In countries near the equator, where it's warmer during the day, a siesta is the answer. But for those who work in a cubicle, the sound of snoring can disrupt a neighbor!

ENERGY BOOSTER

270

Try to resist afternoon sleepiness by shaking up your diet. Maybe a week without caffeine. Or eating a lunch that balances protein with the carbohydrates. Refuse sugary snacks (they sound good when you're tired, but the quick energy boost doesn't last). Try fruit or a protein bar instead.

If you need it, stand up and stretch, change the light in your office, or lay your head down with eyes closed for a few minutes (in the conference room?). Keep your brain-heavy work for a different time of the day.

Appreciate Your Body

You pay attention to your body—you clothe it, feed it, brush its teeth, exercise it, feed it vitamins, put it to bed at night. It gives you energy to move through life. But do you love it? Do you even like it? Loving your body gives you motion and energy during the day. There are many facets to love, and you don't have to be "perfect" first.

Touch your foot, your thigh, your stomach and appreciate its workings, mentally or aloud. Thank you for getting work done. Thank you for breathing. Thank you for getting me here today. Thanking your body can be hard work in an image-conscious society. Some people focus on what they don't like—big hips, stomach full from lunch, fallen arches—before the first "Thank you" is said. Still, thank your body for its breathing, digesting, hugging.

Take the thanks in front of a mirror. Thank you, or I love you. Those words melt criticisms about how you should look and act. Life with fewer of those injunctions helps you act from what you—not what readers of *Vogue* magazine—really need.

Worry Less

Face it: We worry. It's part of being human. Trying to get somewhere in our lives, knowing we're not in control, and fretting over details. Worry is a toned-down form of fear. It doesn't necessarily take over our daily lives, but it nags like a backseat driver. Constant worry is our mind in spasm. And it wastes our energy.

Worry may be a human trait, but we can slow it down and take back our lives. Noticing is the first step. Dr. Edward Hallowell in *Worry: Controlling It and Using It Wisely* suggests some other ways:

1. Educate yourself about the problem and ramifications.
2. Talk usefully to yourself—is there some action you can take?
3. Connect to others; connect to a higher spiritual sense.
4. Move your body—breathe, walk, stretch.
5. If needed, try therapy or medication.

And since nothing lasts forever (even worry), imagine yourself happily through the situation.

Create Ministructures

Our minds are filled with details that occupy a lot of brain space—passwords, PINs at the ATM, the welcome screen on the cell phone. These are usually routine messages or a series of numbers or letters to enter—a birthday, street address, number of nephews.

However, you can do more with these detailed parts of your life. You can use them to remind yourself of clues to what you really want. These ministructures can help your unconscious mind remember simple tasks or new places to grow.

For instance: Perhaps you want to feel more love in your life. Having a great relationship may be the best picture, but the feeling you crave is being loved. Change your computer password to "I feel loved" and see if you notice that coworkers or your sisters or children really do love you. Or what if you want to write ten to twenty pages a day on your novel? Make your ATM pin number 1020. If your welcome screen on your computer says a boring, "Hello, Esmerelda" and it makes you feel robotic, change it to "Esmerelda, you knock my socks off!" and feel a tinge of glee. When these messages or passwords become just a routine part of your inner life, change them again—add a new goal! Use the structure of your machine-filled existence to make your life sing.

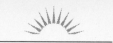

Meditate on Your Coffee or Tea

How much do you love your coffee or tea? Maybe you drink it daily. You love how it gets you going. You put in exactly the condiments right for you—a half-teaspoon of sugar and some nonfat milk. But do you really pay attention to the coffee or tea itself? A mini-meditation on your drink can wake you like the caffeine or herbs themselves.

Give yourself five—or even fifteen—minutes in this moment of awareness, from Lorin Roche's *Meditation Made Easy*. Sit in a comfortable spot with your hot drink. Hold the warmth in your fingers. Breathe in the misty aroma drifting above the cup. Close your eyes and become aware of your body's response. Is you mouth watering? Does your belly react? After several long moments, prepare to take a taste. Notice your hands lifting, your mouth opening, the warmth on your lips. Can you feel the hot liquid on your tongue, the heat in your throat or belly? Is it bitter, sweet, fatty, tangy?

Before you finish the whole cup, hold it again in your hands. Breathe in the sensations you just experienced. Each sip, try being aware of many moments. And come back to the drink when your mind meanders away. When your drinking is full of awareness, you celebrate the art of coffee—and the art of your life.

ENERGY
BOOSTER

274

Lend a Hand

Some days, lack of energy feels blue, alone, all given out. Life becomes the stuff you do, not your real self. We think we need to take more in—a massage, a nice meal, pampering. Taking in is wonderful, but it can still leave us missing something. Missing the zing in giving out.

Lending a hand—volunteering—means gaining a new sense of purpose in your life. It means expanding your community, your skills, your belonging to the larger world. It fills the balance of your life beyond the everyday.

Where to volunteer? An animal shelter? Homeless shelter? With children or the elderly? Write down a short list of what you do that increases your joy. Then call on the volunteer coordinator at United Way, a nursing home, school, shelter, soup kitchen. . . . While talking to the coordinator, notice if you have that sense of joy. Do you think you'd feel helpful, contributing, a part of the larger world? When you find a place that makes your heart sing, spend a few hours a month there for six months. The habit of giving will add meaning, richness, and energy to your own life, too.

Do-It-Yourself Energy Bars

These bars, courtesy of Hershey's kitchen, are loaded with protein to keep you going throughout the day.

1/2 cup butter, softened
1 cup packed light brown
   sugar
2 eggs
1 teaspoon vanilla extract
1/3 cup cocoa powder
1/4 cup low-fat milk
1/4 cup whole wheat flour

1/4 cup nonfat dry milk
   powder
1/4 cup wheat germ
1/2 tsp. baking powder
1/4 tsp. baking soda
1 (10 oz.) package peanut
   butter chips
1/2 cup raisins

Preheat oven to 350° F. Grease 13 x 9 x 2-inch baking pan. In large mixer bowl, beat butter, brown sugar, eggs, and vanilla until light and fluffy. Blend in cocoa and milk. Stir together whole wheat flour, nonfat dry milk powder, wheat germ, baking powder, and baking soda; add to butter mixture, beating until well blended. Stir in peanut butter chips and raisins. Spread batter evenly into prepared pan. Bake 30 to 35 minutes. Cool completely in pan on wire rack. Cut into bars. Makes about 36 brownies.

Jump Rope

Here's one you can do anywhere. If you don't have a rope, pretend you do. Simply jump for one minute as if you were skipping rope. You'll get the old blood circulating and will feel instantly energized.

Put Your Feet Up

Remember as a teenager, that urge to scrunch on a sofa with your feet up? It doesn't disappear once we're adults. Sitting at your desk, even in an ergonomic chair, can cause back and leg pain. A quick and easy response: a footrest.

Good footrests tilt so your toes are higher than your heels. They cause you to sit further back in the chair for better support, and they slightly tip your pelvis into the chair back as well. This helps improve the alignment of your spine, increasing lumbar (lower) back support, and reducing back strain and fatigue when sitting for long periods.

Check out the footrests in office supply and furniture stores, made from wood, metal, and inflatable plastic. Some are adjustable, some help circulation with a gentle rocking motion. Once you start using a footrest, you'll wonder what's missing when you work at a desk that doesn't have one!

Solve Your Problems While You Sleep

While you are engaged in your everyday activities, unsolved problems remain in the back of your mind, awaiting your attention and draining your energy. Your dreams or nightly intuition may be able to help. Just write a short note before you go to sleep asking for information about a sticky situation. You might find the solution in your awareness as you wake up, or it may reveal itself sometime during the day.

Check Your Medicine Cabinet

Many common over-the-counter medicines and prescription drugs cause tiredness. Sleeping pills are obvious, but antihistamines (even the so-called nondrowsy ones), beta-blockers, antidepressants, and antianxiety medicine, as well as blood pressure, seizure, and cholesterol medicine can be making you want to close your eyes.

A friend of ours had no energy whatsoever. It turned out that her cholesterol-lowering medicine was to blame. Her doctor changed the dose, and she's up and about again.

ENERGY
BOOSTER

280

Try Support Stockings

It's easy to take feet and legs for granted. And yet they do so much. Taking us walking, running, or dancing. Ambling up and down the grocery-store aisles. Supporting us at work. Between the effort they make and the gravity of our bodies, legs do a lot of work, especially pumping blood from the toes back to the heart.

Treating feet nicely can make the day go better—especially for those who spend a lot of time either standing or sitting. A great way to support your legs and feet is wearing supporting socks or stockings. They feel tight when they're first on, but during the day or evening, it feels as if you have your own walking masseuse!

The more support you can give your legs and feet, the more they can support your day.

Turn Off Your Television

Seems like a relaxed hour or two on the couch, feet up, soft drink in hand, would be just the ticket to rejuvenation. But what if it's accompanied by flickering colored lights; music, dialogue, and sounds that change at least every ninety seconds; and larger-than-life-sized heads encouraging you to feel hungry, desirous, sad, disgusted, or amused? Would it still be rejuvenating?

ENERGY
BOOSTER

282

When you watch TV, your body is in relaxed repose, and you feel engaged and stimulated. But you're also processing a lot of information. And being asked for a lot of responses— emotional, intellectual, and physical. Television provides virtual company and brain amusement, especially nice for sending mental talk and criticism to the background. But television doesn't often give what we really want: connection to people, or a different view on worries, a gentler way of being with ourselves. (Although it's great for folding laundry!)

See what life is like if you veg out without TV. Turn off your TV regularly—once a week, every day between five and eight o'clock, for a whole week or month—and see what other things you get done that you'd forgotten that you really want to do.

Pine On

The holiday rush got you run down? Sniff a Christmas tree.
Honestly. Apparently there is something in fir and pine that
stimulates a nerve in the nose to release adrenaline. And don't
just give a tiny sniff. Inhale deeply for a minute or two and
notice how much more peppy you feel.

Get Enough Antioxidants

Antioxidants found in vitamins and minerals are the foundation of the body's energy-creating system. They help the body get nutrients, which means they create the conditions under which your body can get the energy from the food you are consuming. (They also have cancer-fighting properties.) They include: vitamin C (recommended dose 500–2000 mg), vitamin E (recommended dose 100–800 IU), CoQ10 (recommended dose 50–150 mg), beta-carotene (recommended dose 15,000 IU), selenium (recommended dose 50–200mg), copper (recommended dose 1.5–3 mg), and manganese (recommended dose 2–5 mg).

How Much Does that Short Cut Cost?

You want to get home. You're tired of work, tired of traffic. The kids, dry cleaning, or both are in the back, dinner needs to be made, you want to put your feet up on the couch already. You've been waiting all day to get home and relax, and this red light is the last obstacle in your way. You could skip over to the side streets instead of waiting for the left arrow to turn green. But will it really benefit you?

Short cuts offer two temptations: a sense of control and the possibility of a little less time on the road. But short cuts aren't free. They can cost in terms of stress (navigating narrower streets with parked cars and kids and dogs running around) and attention (checking the cross streets, left and right, at every corner). And you know that stress and attention can drain your energy. So you end up needing more renewal when you finally make it home.

See how you feel rolling up in front of your home after conniving the best short cuts. Then the next day, experiment with some smooth breathing, shoulder rolls, or even a brief eyes-shut moment at that red light instead. Again, check out your disposition before you head into the house. Maybe you'll find that you've begun your end-of-the-day renewal in the car, saving the price of the short cuts.

Give Something Away

It's been said that each household can give away one grocery bag of unneeded goods a week just to keep pace with all we buy—and that's in addition to garbage! Giving away items that you don't love or can't use (but that are still in good shape) frees up your energy.

You don't have to spend the day, or even an hour, chasing down every last scarf and gravy boat. Simply take a grocery bag or box and go quickly through a closet or room or the house. Give yourself fifteen minutes to find as many things as you can that you no longer want but someone else might. Then close up the bag or box with tape and put it in the trunk of your car.

Where should those things go, charity or a yard sale? Giving items to someone who will use them gratefully makes them more valuable than selling them to a bargain hunter. Plus, do you really want to spend your newly freed energy on running a yard sale? The next time you're out, find a Goodwill box, church, or charitable resale store that can make use of those "useless" items.

Get on Track

When you're tired, your eyes don't track smoothly. That means that someone watching you read would see a slight shimmy as your eyes move from left to right. That shimmy means you might skip words or have a hard time tracking the line you just read. And that adds frustration and inefficiency to reading.

To strengthen your tracking, you need just a pen or pencil. Hold it about eighteen inches in front of your nose, then slowly move it left and then right. Keep your head still and watch it with your eyes. Return to center and track it again, this time up and down. Then track the two diagonals, upper right to lower left and vice versa.

Maybe you'll find that textbook on internal rates of return in actuarial statistics actually readable—or at least less draining!

Crank the High
Energy Tunes

Find yourself flagging in the car? Put on some music with one
beat per second, and you'll soon find yourself bopping along.
And if you sing along, so much the better. Pink, Red Hot Chili
Peppers, No Doubt—whatever gets your energy going.

Pull Your Hair Out

No, not really. This energy booster combines an inversion—a yoga term for putting your heart above your head—a neck release, and scalp stimulation, bringing blood flow to the brain. If you're bald, you may have to skip this one, but you can do the inversion.

With your feet hip-width apart, exhale and curl your spine from your head until you're hanging over. If your hamstrings feel tight, just bend your knees. Near the crown of your head, grab a fistful of hair in each hand and gently pull down. People vary on the sensitivity in their scalp, but you should be able to find a gentle pull that feels good, maybe keeping your palms flat and close to your head as you pull the hair between your fingers.

Can you feel your neck unkink? Take three to five breaths here. When you're ready to rise, first exhale, then slowly come up as you inhale, letting your head hang until the last moment. Standing, feel your spine and tingling scalp grow tall.

Cozy Up to an Indoor Plant

Plants nourish our physical and emotional health. They are color magnets, endless variations on shapes, kinesthetic sculptures that react to passersby. They provide oxygen and moisture for the air we breathe, they reduce dust. Norwegian researchers discovered that indoor plants could lessen fatigue, coughs, and sore throats by more than 30 percent. NASA space research found that ordinary spider plants and peace lilies effectively cleaned the air.

Enter a room with plants, and you feel more welcomed, more relaxed. Even in a low-light office environment with little time for maintenance, you can find plants to work for you. Ask at a garden store for a philodendron, aglaonema, dracaenas (dragon tree), Neanthebella Palm, sansevieria (snake plant), scheffleras (umbrella plant), or a ficus.

Let growing things support your growing.

Eat a Rainbow

Naturally colored fruits and vegetables supply energy to keep you going as well as providing you with many other health benefits. Reds in tomatoes, watermelon, and papaya contain lycopene, an antioxidant to fight cancer. Oranges/yellows provide vitamin C, folate, beta-carotene (boosts the immune system) and carotenoids (to protect the skin and eyes). Green veggies contain minerals, fiber, and antioxidants (in leafy greens). Blues/purples have anthocyanins to protect against carcinogens and may help prevent heart disease. Whites contain allicin, which may help lower cholesterol and blood pressure.

Get a Boost from a Protein Shake

You may be dragging because you're not getting enough protein, which gives sustained energy. You can try protein powder, but many people hate the taste. The recipe below offers ten grams of protein and is loaded with iron to boot!

$^1/_3$ cup chopped dates softened in $^3/_4$ cup almond
    or soy milk
$^1/_2$ cup nonfat plain yogurt
$^1/_2$ cup soft tofu
2 tbs. tahini
1 banana, sliced

Place all ingredients in a blender and whir until smooth. Makes about three cups.

Brush Your Shoulders

Energy gets congested in the tension of your shoulders. An invigorating idea is using a hairbrush to break up that congestion and free your liveliness, from Donna Eden's *Energy Medicine.*

Take a hairbrush (use whatever you have at hand, but if you like this technique you may want to buy a stiff-bristled brush at the drug store) and tap your shoulders with it. Use a steady rhythm to help the tension dissipate. Do both shoulders. When you're done, relish the tingle that replaces the numbness.

Eliminate Glare

We spend a lot of time processing with our eyes, so when they work too hard, we work too hard. Glare—reflected, harsh light—makes us strain to see our computers or TV screens, puts faces of coworkers in shadow, bounces off the reading page so the black font disappears, makes us squint when we're driving. It causes headaches, eyestrain, fatigue, lack of concentration.

ENERGY
BOOSTER

294

Sometimes we adjust to the glare in our visual surroundings and don't even know it. But we can conserve energy by adjusting the surroundings instead.

You don't have to become a fanatic to adjust glare. Outdoors use polarized sunglasses. Indoors you can move your seat, close the blinds, or add ambient light (like from floor lamps aimed at the ceiling) to diffuse the glare—and the strain on your eyes.

Try an Energy Medicine Healer

In the past decade or so, energy medicine has become increasingly accepted as a valid medical tool. It treats both the physical and energy body by freeing up blocked energy so that healing can occur. Techniques include acupuncture, homeopathy, qigong, therapeutic touch, reiki, and energy psychiatry. To make sure you are getting bona fide treatment, make sure your practitioner is associated with the American Holistic Medical Association or other professional organization with qualifying standards. If you do choose one of these treatments, you should see some upsurge in energy within three weeks. If not, chances are it's not right for you.

Manage Your (and Others')
Holiday Expectations

No, you don't have to be the perfect party hostess. Or have the best decorated Christmas tree or the perfect colored Easter eggs. Or run all over town for the best presents or cards for those on your list. Holidays are about love and connection. And how available can you be if you can't drag yourself out of bed?

ENERGY
BOOSTER

296

Right now, think about what you want to make happen at holiday time. For each of us it is something different—a great meal together; a relaxing, unstructured time; a few great presents. Then make it clear to friends and family that you are going to do that and nothing else. When you remember what really matters about the holidays for you, you can preserve your energy for those efforts.

Do "Resistive Scheduling"

Resistive scheduling is a phrase coined by Dr. Vern Cherewatenko in his book *The Stress Cure* to refer to "the conscious effort not to fill up every little time slot in the day but to leave buffer room for the unexpected."

You know what he's talking about—things happen. You chip a tooth, the dog has to make an emergency trip to the vet, your computer crashes. If we schedule ourselves to fill every minute of every day, when these unexpected emergencies arise, we have to spend a tremendous amount of time and energy to deal with them.

If, however, we schedule room in our day for the unexpected, we can deal with these minor irritations with a minimum of energy expenditure.

Follow Your Passions

Your passions—what you love to do—are part of what make you unique. They seemingly come out of nowhere and possess you; after all, how else can you explain one person's love of fly fishing, another's of raising show dogs, and someone else's of collecting Wedgwood china? To call them hobbies trivializes them and negates the commitment and enjoyment such things represent to each of us. No matter what you call them, all of us have certain things that get our juices flowing, and the more we know what they are and build them into our lives, the more energy we will experience.

What are yours? What do you love to do that perhaps you take for granted—woodworking, quilting, reading cooking magazines, swimming, biking? If you can't think of anything, ask yourself: If there were no constraints of money, time, or other people's opinions and I could do anything, what would I want to do? Once you identify your passions, make a plan to fold at least one into your day, your week, your month.

Pop Some Zinc

Many folks swear by zinc in strengthening the immune system and warding off colds and flus. But zinc is also known for boosting mental alertness. It is found in meat, liver, eggs, and seafood, particularly oysters. Experts believe that as many as 75 percent of Americans are zinc deficient and cannot get the recommended amount in diet alone. If you want to up your zinc level, the recommended daily amount is twenty to thirty milligrams.

Energy and Your Weight

Experts now say that two-thirds of Americans are overweight (as measured by a Body Mass Index BMI of 25 or higher) and one-third are obese (BMI of 30 or higher). No wonder we're so tired. Carrying around all that extra weight is exhausting.

If you are overweight, you are at risk for diabetes, heart disease, stroke, high blood pressure, high cholesterol, gallbladder disease, osteoarthritis, sleep apnea and other breathing problems, and some forms of cancer (uterine, breast, colorectal, kidney, and gallbladder). And you know what it takes to turn the situation around—eat less and exercise more. Ask anyone who's lost the weight—the physical and emotional energy you gain is its own reward.

Eat Throughout the Day

Maybe you wilt because your blood sugar is low. To find out, try eating small, frequent meals throughout the day rather than three big meals and notice how your energy levels change. (You may lose weight too—new diet research shows this approach can be useful in weight control as well.) The trick is to eat before your blood sugar levels dip.

Juice It

Many folks swear by the enlivening effects of fresh vegetable and fruit juices. Depending on what you use, juice from fresh fruits—berries, especially—and vegetables can provide many antioxidants as well as other vitamins, minerals, and fiber. Plus the taste is light and refreshing. Folks who juice claim that they help counteract the harmful effects of caffeine, alcohol, nicotine, and other bad substances. You need a good quality juicer and very fresh fruits and vegetables, preferably organic. You can experiment with various combinations yourself or use a book such as *Juicing for Life* by Cherie Calbom and Maureen Keane.

ENERGY
BOOSTER

302

Bring Your Brain into Balance

Here's a hemisphere-balancing exercise from kinesiology designed to freshen your mind in the middle of the workday. It comes from *Energize Your Life* by Nic Rowley.

1. Stand, feet together, eyes closed, with your arms at shoulder height out to the sides, palms forward.
2. Slowly bring your arms together until your palms meet—keep trying if this does not happen first time—it's more difficult than you might think. Link your fingers and imagine that you are joining the two sides of your brain.
3. Bring your hands in to your chest as if you are drawing in your whole self. Rest with one hand on top of the other.
4. Relax, hands by your sides, eyes closed, and enjoy the calm, satisfied feeling of your brain being in balance.

Do a Random Act of Kindness

We all know what this is—a little something nice for someone else done anonymously: feeding a parking meter, leaving a bouquet, bussing someone else's table at the deli. When we do such things, we feel good about ourselves and the world at large—and that gives us an energy spurt. And chances are we've made someone else's day or hour a bit happier and less stressful too. An added plus: Because an act like this is something easy, it takes very little energy to do.

ENERGY
BOOSTER

304

Eliminate One or More Activities

Are you or your kids overscheduled? Recently Susannah found that she was running her daughter around three nights a week—to ballet, dog training, and piano lessons—on top of a full work schedule and a weekend full of commitments. She and her daughter were often tired and crabby. So they sat down and decided to cut something out. Not because it wasn't good, but because too much of all these good things was exhausting.

Life these days presents so many options and we can get spread so thin that we end up empty vessels. Sometimes the wisest thing to do is to stop doing something pleasurable or educational or enriching, in favor of creating more downtime.

Spend a Day in Bed

When you've been going full speed and your internal gas meter is on empty, how about taking one day on the weekend and just staying in bed? You don't have to sleep—read a good novel or indulge in your favorite magazines, watch mindless TV, indulge in takeout. There's something about being recumbent for a whole twenty-four hours that is really restorative!

Stop Trying to Live Up to Others' Expectations

Do you ever feel that the world is asking too much of you? Chances are it is! Everyone is overloaded, and so anyone who comes along will probably be giving you more to do. At work or at home, we're all looking to offload our burdens onto someone else and/or find someone to make our dreams come true.

When we constantly look outside ourselves for validation, we are at the particular mercy of other people's expectations. And so we will be asked to do more and more, we will take on more and more, and burn out. When we understand we "can't please all of the people all of the time" and the number one person we must please is ourselves by having enough energy to do the things we want to in our lives, we can learn to say without guilt or shame, "I'm sorry if you are disappointed, but I did my best" or "I just can't take that on right now, sorry." We each have only finite energy. Living up to what we expect of ourselves is challenge enough. Don't add other people's expectations to your narrow shoulders.

Choose Where to Focus
Your Energy Today

Attention is energy. Rather than being at the beck and call of everyone at work, like a kite in the wind that has no string, decide where you are going to put your attention for the day or the hour and do not allow interruptions during that time. Tell folks you are on a conference call, close the door, don't check e-mail or answer the phone. Or set up "office hours" in which you make yourself available to all and sundry, like professors do.

When you are conscientious about preserving blocks of time to focus on what you decide you want to do at work, you free up tremendous amounts of energy for the task at hand. (Plus you get more done than if you are in perpetual emergency response, fire-putting-out mode.) The fires will still be there when you open the door again, but you will feel great at all you've chosen to accomplish.

Change the Pictures and Colors on Your Computer

Ever notice that when you flirt with a new lover, your body tingles when you first hold hands? Then after ten minutes you almost forget you're touching. Same process happens with most new experiences: Our bodies eventually get used to and turn off the stimulation.

We might shop for fashionable shoes or the hottest camera to get that "new" charge again. But without spending money—using the technology of computers—you can make subtle changes that charge you up.

You can change colors or pictures on your computer to liven your desk time. The colors of your window borders can turn from classic blues to bold contrasts. Put on a new desktop picture—a landscape or planets spinning or a picture of your family on vacation at the beach. It's easy using the Display menu in the Control Panel—or ask a geeky friend to help you redecorate your desk view. A new picture of flowers or flying toasters can liven you up for a while. When that grows old, you can change it again.

Visualize Energy

Here is a practice from Nic Rowley's *Energize Your Life*. It's called Cook's Hook-up.

1. Standing with both feet planted firmly on the ground, cross your right leg over your left leg and your right arm over your left arm; now link fingers together.
2. Keeping your fingers locked, twist your hands under and up, and at the same time press your tongue to the roof of your mouth. Breathe deeply, and visualize energy flowing around your body for one minute.
3. Keeping your tongue pressed into the roof of your mouth, uncross your arms and legs. Stand with your feet apart, bend your arms up and touch fingertips, then breathe deeply for one minute. Repeat the whole sequence, this time crossing your left leg over your right leg and your left arm over your right arm.

Treat Yourself

Sometimes you just need to indulge yourself a little so that your whole life doesn't feel like drudgery. What would be a good treat for you right now? A manicure? Massage? Buying that necklace you've been eyeing for weeks in the jewelry store? A makeover? What would bring a smile to your face and a spring to your step? Go for something that will perk you up without breaking the bank and causing money worries later.

Solve Your Problems While You Sleep

While you're involved in your everyday activities, unsolved problems can remain in the back of your mind, awaiting your attention and draining your energy. Your dreams or nightly intuition may be able to help. Just write a short note before you sleep asking for information about a sticky situation. You might find the solution in your awareness as you wake up, or it may reveal itself sometime during the day.

Train Properly

In their book *The Power of Full Engagement*, Jim Loehr and Tony Swartz explain how managing our energy rather than our time is the key to high performance and self-renewal. They use a secret that high performance athletes in training know—namely that you must work very hard (what they call extension) and take time to recover or else you aren't working at your peak. If you don't extend enough, you never build up muscle; if you don't recover, you keep tearing down the muscle you just built up.

They have created a system by which you incorporate extension and recovery in the four domains of your life—physical, mental, emotional, and spiritual. Here's a way to begin to think about this for yourself. What are your extension (pushing yourself to new heights) and recovery (rest and renewal) in the physical domain? In the mental? In the emotional? In the spiritual? Each of us has ways we exert ourselves and recover; they are different for us all. One person's recovery strategy in physical, say yoga, may be another person's spiritual extension. There are no wrong answers. Now rank yourself in each category of both extension and recovery on a scale of 1 to 10, 1 being doing it very little, 10 doing it a lot.

Where do you need to train more? Perhaps your life has gotten a bit stale and you need more mental exertion. Or you're not doing any emotional recovery. The more you are in balance between extension and recovery in the four domains, the more energy you'll have.

Eat a Good Breakfast

It's easy to skip breakfast, especially when you're in a hurry. And inner hunger doesn't always get up steam until you've started moving through your day. You get coffee and a Danish, then wonder why you're dreary at ten a.m.

Brains need some glucose to function (not sugar, but digested food)—and in the morning, there's not a lot of glucose up there. To keep the body going through the day, it's good to have some protein and fiber. You know the routine—a bowl of cereal, oatmeal, eggs. For rushed mornings, a protein shake (or smoothie) can be made the night before. In the morning, shake it up and drink it as you sort the e-mail and check the day's to-do list.

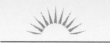

Don't Be Afraid to Slow Down

Some of us have no energy because we never slow down. We're stressaholics, workaholics, whatever you want to call it; we can't ever seem to stop and recharge our batteries. You know who you are—you haven't taken a vacation in years, you work almost every weekend, you get in early to the office and leave late. And you always have a good reason: a big client meeting, a crisis at work, a push project. But the emergencies never end.

Fundamentally you are afraid to take a break and recharge because you would then have to feel your emotions: anger, fear, loneliness, sadness—the whole 10,000 sorrows, as the Buddhists call them. And as long as you keep moving, you don't have to feel them.

But you pay a price, a big price, for this avoidance. You run a very great risk of complete mental, emotional, and physical energy burnout. The Chinese character for busy is a combination of the characters for heart and death—meaning staying busy will ultimately kill you. Do you need to get to that point before you do something about this constant depletion of energy? One workaholic told us recently, "I'm secretly hoping for a heart attack or something that will not kill me, but will force me to stop." If this description fits you, be honest with yourself. Tell yourself the truth of why you can't stop. Then find help to bring you back into balance—therapy, coaching, or talks with a trusted friend.

Learn How You Focus Your Attention

In a meeting or a class, do you feel your energy sagging? Do you feel spaced out? Maybe your brain is being triggered into producing more alpha and theta waves. So suggests Dawna Markova in her book, *The Open Mind*. In it, she explains that when we're awake, our brains are producing three types of waves: beta, alpha, and theta. Beta is the state of mind when you are paying attention externally, where it is the easiest to focus on what's going on around you. Alpha is a state of mind when you are aware of both external and internal—you know that something's happening outside you and you are aware of your inner state of mind as well. Theta is when you are paying attention completely inwardly and lose touch with your surroundings. For each of us, something triggers these states of mind—for some, talking produces more beta waves; for others, moving does; for still others, looking or writing does. Ditto for the other two brainwave states.

If you find your mind wandering and less sharp when you have to sit for long periods of time and listen and talk, chances are if you take notes (visual) or fiddle with a pencil, beads, or playdough (moving) for instance, your energy will stay more focused and alert.

Manage Your Chronic Pain

Millions of us suffer from chronic pain—and for those of you who have never experienced it, it can sap your energy and consume your whole life. Folks used to have to suffer in silence, but no more. Pain management is now a medical specialty and it *can* be treated. In fact, it's very important if you are suffering from any kind of chronic pain, whatever the cause, to get aggressive treatment as soon as possible. Otherwise, in a process known as deconditioning your body gets used to feeling that way and it is harder to treat. For help in your area, visit the Web site for the American Academy of Pain Management at *www.aapainmanage.org*.

Work from Your Strengths

Recent research of two million people around the world by the Gallup organization discovered that each of us has five or six core thinking talents, ways of thinking that we have done since we were very young that by the time we become adults have created deep "grooves" in our brain. The more we understand what these are, the more we can use them on purpose and do work that aligns with our talents. Why this is important is that the more that we use these talents, the more energy we have and the less we burn out. That's because it's easy for us to think in this particular way because the neuropathways are so strong. When we have to think in other ways, we can force ourselves to do it, but it takes a lot of energy.

To learn more, you can read *Now Discover Your Strengths* and take the Gallup on-line assessment. Or you can take a similar self assessment offered on Martin Seligman's *www.auth entichappiness.org* Web site.

Practice Gratitude

As an experiment, notice how you feel right now on a scale of 1 to 10, 1 being the worst ever and 10 being absolutely fabulous. What's your number? Now think of everything that is wrong with you and your life and how awful you feel. Now what's your number? Chances are it went down. Now think of all that you have to be grateful for in your life, all the blessings you've received and continue to receive. Really take time to count them. Now what's your number. It went up, right?

Gratitude is an amazing energy booster because it focuses our attention on all that is good and right with us and our world, and we become filled with joy, hope, and optimism, which are powerful mental and spiritual energetic states.

There are many ways to practice—keeping a gratitude journal, contemplating blessings before bed, saying thanks before eating. Whatever works for you is just fine. And during the day, when you start to flag, taking a moment to notice the good in your life will perk you right up.

Receive the Energy of Others

Do you allow yourself to receive the energy of others? It comes in many forms—offers to help, compliments, presents, a smile at just the right moment. Many of us have trouble receiving, though, and therefore we don't take in these wonderful gifts in a way that they can be experienced and benefited from. Susannah recently found herself flicking off praise and an invitation to lunch, thinking to herself, "Oh, she doesn't really mean it."

ENERGY
BOOSTER

320

Do you block yourself from receiving the upward lift you can get from others? Do you never ask for help? Dismiss offers to assist you? If you find yourself drained at the end of every day, chances are you do. What would happen if you started the day by asking yourself, I wonder what I will receive today—from other people, from the universe. The more you notice, the more you'll be buoyed up.

Check Your Motivation

In his book *The Path of Least Resistance*, Robert Fritz identifies two orientations toward life. He calls them creative and reactive. In a creative orientation, you are seeking to bring something new into existence because you want to. Your motivation is internal, you feel compelled to act from an inner source of power. When you come from a reactive orientation, you act to get rid of or avoid something. You are motivated externally, by circumstances outside yourself that you want to get away from.

We can do anything from either orientation, if only we know which. For instance, we can write a book to get rid of debt or we can write it to bring new ideas into being. Why does our motivation matter? Because, says Fritz, a creative orientation is endlessly sustainable because you literally create energy from the act of bringing something into being. A reactive orientation, on the other hand, drains energy and is not sustainable over a long period of time. It's the difference between having a solar generator inside yourself and a battery that will run down. Where in your life are you motivated from a creative orientation? If you can find and follow that, your energy levels will soar.

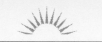

Do a Solar Plexus Tune Up

According to Eastern medicine, the chakras are the seven major centers of the body's energy system that penetrate the aura and the physical body. The solar plexus chakra, located in the upper abdomen, regulates the digestive tract and is associated with power, potential, will, prosperity, drive, and ambition. One of the symptoms of a blockage here is fatigue, a loss of power, will, drive. To tune up this area, try this meditation by Dr. Brenda Davies in *Chakra Power Beads*: Get into a comfortable position and

> *take a deep breath . . . letting anything negative flow out of the soles of your feet. . . . Take another deep breath, and this time breathe in white light through the top of your head; allow it to shine through every cell. . . . Take your attention to your solar plexus. Breathe gently into it and . . . visualize it opening to reveal bright yellow light, like the midday sun. Feel its energy spreading through you, filling you with power. See yourself as the powerful, mighty being you are, capable of fulfilling your potential, being successful and living a prosperous life. . . . Feel every cell tingle as your energy moves powerfully. You are healing and being energized while you remain grounded and aware of your humanity. You are ready to face life and any challenge with optimism and courage. . . . With a breath, ask your solar plexus to close, holding its power within you . . . gently open your eyes.*

ENERGY
BOOSTER

322

Use a Mantra

When things are swirling faster and faster, you can use a mantra, a word or phrase that you say to remind you to keep your center and therefore conserve your energy. In her book *Positive Energy*, Judith Orloff explains that one way to translate the word mantra is "that which protects you from negative energy." It's a way not to get caught up in a downward spiral of energy-draining negativity.

Find one that works for you. In her book *The Power of Patience*, M. J. Ryan suggests: "I have all the time I need." Orloff suggests the Beatles' "Let it be." It doesn't matter what it is, as long as it works to increase your positive energy. You can say it silently or out loud, and you might want to write it somewhere where you can see it whenever you need it.

Set Clear Boundaries

How much of your energy goes into doing things you don't want to do because you were afraid to say no, or rehashing things over and over with someone, particularly a child, because you haven't set limits in such a way that it's nonnegotiable? If so, you need to learn how to set clear boundaries and stick to them. The energy you will save as a consequence will be astounding.

Step one: Tell yourself the truth about what is acceptable and unacceptable to you in a given situation. Do you really want to host the in-laws for two full weeks? Is it okay with you if your son stays up till ten p.m.? This is crucial; if you don't know what's true for you, you can't enforce anything.

Next, explain what's true for you: "I'm looking forward to your visit, but I have a project due that second week so since I want us all to really enjoy one another, it would be better if you came only for one week." Or, "You must be in bed by nine; otherwise you can't get up in the morning." If you get protests, flak, or push-back, you can always say, "I understand that you feel differently," or "I'm sorry you don't agree, but that's what's true for me, so I'm sticking with it." You may have to repeat yourself several times, but if you stand solidly yet kindly on your point, chances are the other will pick up on your refusal to waver and respect it.

Understand Your Energy Habits

For each of us, our life force manifests in four kinds of energy: mental, emotional, physical, and spiritual. And they are not separate—each profoundly affects the others. Each also is associated with a particular element. Your physical energy is earth energy. Emotional energy is associated with water—tears, overflowing feelings. Mental energy corresponds to the air, the energy of consciousness, while fire—passion, commitment—is associated with spiritual energy.

Each of us has a particular energy habit, a way of relying on certain of these energies when we face obstacles or challenges in our lives. Some of us are very "fiery," responding passionately to almost everything. Others use air strategies, becoming very mental or analytic. Others overflow with feelings (water); still others get very stubborn and unmoving (earth). What is your primary energy habit? Do you use them all? Do you over-rely on one? In what situations do you use which? The more we become conscious about these energies, the more choice we have to use one or another, where appropriate.

Stay Away from Refined Sugar

Foods with lots of refined sugar sure taste good. And they do give you an immediate burst of energy. But that burst comes with a high price—an energetic crash an hour or so later. So if you want to avoid the sugar blues, stay away from desserts and sugary snacks and try fruit instead.

ENERGY
BOOSTER

326

Refresh Your Eyes

Our eyes are often the first indicator of fatigue. They can feel sleepy and sensitive even when our bodies have vigor. Our eyes are constantly subject to strain in this world: driving, computer work, TV viewing, reading, and even walking through a crowd. Recharging your eyes can free your body to use its energy on other things.

Palming is a great way to refresh your eyes. Simply rest your elbows on the table and place your cheekbones on the heels of your hands. Then cup your hands over your eyes and place the top of the palms on your eyebrows. Block as much light as possible. Now close your eyes. Let yourself imagine something very, very dark, like black velvet. The dark will let your eyes naturally dilate and rest. Imagine your breath going to the muscles and membranes of your eyes to relax them further. When you are ready to stop, open your eyes, blink a few times, and remove your hands from your face. You'll be surprised how much easier it is to function when your eyes are happy.

Vacate for at Least a Week

Want to know why we're all so tired? We're working more—100 hours per couple per year as compared to twenty years ago—and taking less time off. We work more hours than even the Japanese, who coined the term for sudden death in men: "death by overwork." Americans have never been too liberal with time off, even when we take it. According to the U.S. Bureau of Labor statistics, the average worker gets one to two weeks paid vacation; if you've been with a company twenty years, you will have crept up to three. Contrast that with Europe where everyone gets five to six weeks of paid time off!

All this work is not good. We never get a chance to recharge our batteries in any significant way. Research shows that it takes at least a week to ten days of vacation to be replenished and restored. So skimping on time off isn't smart. You'll end up making more mistakes and taking more time to get less done.

When was the last time you had a vacation? Expense is no excuse—you can stay home. As long as you really don't work—no e-mails, work phone calls, etc.—it should do you a world of good.

Change Your Environment

Those who study energy claim that the objects in your environment carry the energy of the people associated with those things. So it's important when you want to change your own energy to clear your home of things associated with circumstances you are trying to change or people you are trying to leave behind. Perhaps you don't want the file cabinet from that failed business in your office. Perhaps you should not wear the watch from that relationship that went bad. Go around your home and office looking at your objects in that way and clear out anything associated with bad or negative energy. Then notice how that makes you feel.

Let Go of Grudges

When we hold onto negative feelings about people or circumstances, we tie up our energy in anger, bitterness, and regret. When we practice forgiveness, in contrast, we free up our bodies, minds, and spirits to experience greater vitality and aliveness. This doesn't mean, especially in the case of terrible wrongs such as abuse, that we deny what happened to us. We choose forgiveness not because the perpetrator necessarily deserves it, but because we want to move on.

Before we can forgive, however, we must heal by acknowledging the grievance and grieving the wound. At some point in this process of emotional resolution, however, there comes time for forgiveness, which moves us out of the victim stance.

Are you holding on to something you are ready to let go of?

Make Snap Decisions

If you find yourself spending a great deal of energy on decision making, perhaps you are going about it in the wrong way. Rather than going back and forth, try making a snap decision by tuning in to your intuition.

Everyone experiences intuition differently. For some folks it's a feeling in their chests, one for yes and another for no. For others, it's a picture that comes into their minds. For others, a feeling in the gut. Or the hair on the back of their necks stands up. Or a voice in their ear. There are as many signals as there are people, and you may have several signals.

Practice tuning in to those signals and acting upon them. If that feels too drastic, try living with the decision for a day and notice how that seems. If it doesn't seem right in twenty-four hours, try something else. The mental energy you save will be enormous.

Discover Your Optimum Break Pattern

In *The Energy Edge*, sports nutritionist Pamela Smith suggests that to optimize energy, we need to take frequent work breaks: "More breaks, more breakthroughs." But she notes that many of us don't take the breaks we need to. In order to figure out what works for you, ask yourself the following questions from her book:

What kind of work exhausts you the most?
What kind of work invigorates you?
How long a period can you work at your best?
What kinds of breaks leave you refreshed?
What kinds of breaks leave you unfocused, distracted, even disoriented?
How do you procrastinate taking breaks?
What is your attitude about breaks?
How do you work best?

Now, look at your answers and schedule breaks in your day around what you've discovered.

Run from Energy Vampires

You know who we're talking about—those folks that seem to sap your energy just being in their presence. They do it through their negativity about everything—how much they've been victimized, how you aren't okay, how nothing will ever work out and you shouldn't even try. Pretty soon you're down in the dumps with them, too tired to even put up a fight.

To preserve your energy, you can distance yourself from these people as much as possible. If for some reason that's not possible—it's a relative you see often, for instance—you can tell them you choose to look at things differently because looking on the gloomy side isn't energizing. Or you can disarm them with kindness and positivism: "Thanks for sharing. I'm holding out the hope that you'll feel better soon," for instance.

What if the energy vampire is you? First you need to become aware of your negativity. Then you need to see that you have a choice—to continue to bring yourself and everyone in your vicinity down by gossiping, judgmental thinking, and pessimism, or begin to choose to focus on what's good and possible in your life.

Fiddle with Pencils, Beads, or Other Objects

Everyone knows that under stress we go into a fight, flight, or freeze mode (although recent research has discovered that women have another option—affiliate, which is to get together with other women and commiserate) when our hearts start pounding, blood flows to our core, and our bodies are flooded with adrenaline. But did you know that because so many of us are under such chronic stress that the adrenaline response can be on almost all the time? No wonder we're pooped out; this response was designed to be on only in emergencies.

One way to reduce the tension and therefore turn the fight or flight response off, says Robert E. Thayer in *Calm Energy*, is to slowly twirl a pencil or toothpick, or very slowly tap your foot or fingers in a way that relaxes the muscles. Or take a short walk, purposely concentrating on relaxing your muscles. Or take several deep breaths, relaxing your muscles as you breathe out. The more we get out of fight or flight, the less tired we'll feel.

ENERGY
BOOSTER

334

Give a Sincere Compliment

Go ahead—make someone's day with a heartfelt compliment on something you admire or appreciate about them. Not only will he or she get a lift, but you will too—the act of appreciation itself increases our joie de vivre.

Think Less

Thinking is a great tool for breaking down problems, for asking big questions, for learning facts. But when the situation needs creative problem solving or intuitive awareness, too much thinking is a waste of energy. Like pounding on a nail head with the butt of a screwdriver. To understand the difference between thinking and awareness, try this experiment: Think about the back of your right knee. . . . Think about your chin. . . . Think about your heart. . . . Now: Become aware of the back of your right knee. Become aware of your chin. Become aware of your heart. Did you sense a difference?

ENERGY BOOSTER

336

With thinking, a part of your brain is concentrating on penetrating a problem. With awareness, your mind and body absorb information on a different scale. If you're in the midst of an exhausting life cycle, like a career change, try thinking about it less. Instead, before you fall asleep or right after you awaken, become aware of your dilemma as if you were viewing it from afar or holding it in your heart. Let some solutions or directions arise from this awareness. Then use your thinking tool to figure out how to make those solutions work. You'll use less energy when you have the whole toolbox in your brain to use.

Use Eucalyptus Oil in the Shower

The strong scent of eucalyptus is great for a mental perk-up. It increases blood flow to the brain, which gives the old gray matter more oxygen, and triggers the brain chemicals epinephrine and norepinephrine, which all means more energy. Get some essential oil and apply it to a washcloth that's been soaked in hot water. Or try Dr. Bronner's Eucalyptus liquid soap. Breathe deeply. If you have a steam shower, put it into the stream of steam for a real head rush!

Become Ergonomically Correct

When you sit at the computer all day, you can easily exhaust yourself. Make sure your feet are flat on the floor when you are sitting at your desk, with your back straight, and your head level with your monitor. Your hands should rest comfortably on the keyboard with your elbows bent at ninety degrees. If you are typing from a book or reading material, prop it up so that you don't have to bend your head to read it. And make sure your font size is large enough to prevent eyestrain!

ENERGY
BOOSTER

338

Do Something "Bad"

Maybe you have low energy because you are stuck in a responsibility rut, being so good at crossing things off your to-do list that you feel half dead. When was the last time you did something different, just for the hell of it—ran barefoot on the "no trespassing" beach, put purple streaks in your hair? Or didn't do something you were "supposed" to do—skipped out on an obligatory dinner, played hooky from work?

If you pride yourself on being a "good" girl or boy, maybe you need to shake yourself up a bit by behaving atypically. This is not permission to cause harm to a person or thing, including yourself. Just an invitation to go intentionally a little wild, to defy convention or your preconceived self-image. Like a friend of ours who went to a Rolling Stone's concert on a motorcycle at the age of seventy-five. Her kids were horrified, but she was energized for weeks!

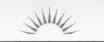

Take Your Vites with OJ

Researchers at Cornell University have discovered that you can maximize the amount of iron in your blood stream—and therefore feel less tired—if you take your iron supplement or multivitamin with an acidic drink, such as orange or grapefruit juice.

Drink Red Tea

Red tea will perk you right up because it has more caffeine than other types of caffeinated teas. But it still has much less than coffee! Available at fine tea shops.

Get Moving First Thing in the Morning

"Morning activity sends a signal to your brain that it's time to kick into gear and helps reset your internal clock," says Thomas Kilkenny, MD, director of the Sleep Apnea Center at Staten Island University Hospital in New York, in an article in *Natural Health* magazine. To boot up your body in the morning, Kilkenny suggests an energizing yoga technique known as Standing Swings. Stand with your feet hip distance apart and your arms at your sides. Turn your torso from side to side, gently swinging your arms so they slap lightly against your body. As you turn, look over the shoulder you're swinging toward and lift the opposite heel. Inhale through your nose as you turn to the front and exhale through your mouth as you swing to the side. Continue to swing for a couple of minutes.

Make a Won't-Do List

Everyone has a to-do list, that seemingly never ending track-ing system of things that you must absolutely get done. So how about freeing yourself from its tyranny by creating a won't-do list as well—those things that you can't or choose not to get to this week? By getting them off your task list, you give your-self a bit of mental relief and take more control of what you do with your time. You can always consult your won't-do list next week to see if you want to put some items over into to-dos. But be sure that there are items going the other direction as well. When you consciously choose to not tackle certain things, you'll feel a lot better about not getting them done and you'll con-serve energy for the really important things in your life.

Sleep on the Right Mattress

You need your beauty rest to feel your best. And maybe you are sleeping on a mattress that's not right for you, that could be seriously impeding your capacity to get your needed Zs. There are so many options out there, from water and air beds to foam, cotton, and other fancy mattresses. Try some out and ask about features. Don't forget to bring your partner along.

ENERGY
BOOSTER

344

Take a Sabbatical

So, you've done a number of suggestions in this book and you are still dragging. Perhaps you need an extended period of time off from your life. Perhaps you need a sabbatical. It's a chance to really recharge your batteries, remember what really matters to you, and help you decide whether to change your life permanently. Academics do it—why can't the rest of us?

If this sounds tempting but you can't figure out how to do it, check out Hope Dlugozima's book *Six Months Off: How to Plan, Negotiate and Take the Break You Need without Burning Bridges or Going Broke*. Maybe you don't even need six months; a couple weeks might just do it. See *Clarity Quest: How to Take A Sabbatical without Taking More Than a Week Off* by Pamela Ammondson.

Let Yourself Off the Hook

Sometimes we're worn out because we blame and guilt-trip ourselves endlessly—it's our fault that our child didn't get into swimming lessons, that our boss didn't say hello to us in the hall, that our friend hasn't called us back. If you're someone who always blames him or herself when things go wrong, try this tip from M. J. Ryan's book *Trusting Yourself.* "Use the psychological technique of re-attribution to expand your thinking. Ask yourself, what other factors could have contributed to this situation besides me?" The pool cut back on lessons; my boss is a jerk; my friend is out of town. Get yourself off the guilt hook and feel your emotional batteries recharging.

Change Negative Energy Patterns

Do you attract the same negative situations over and over? If so, you can free yourself through a process described in *The First Element* by Tae Yun Kim. Begin by looking at something you don't like that's happening in your life right now. See where it has happened before. Then put the pattern into one or two sentences. For instance: "No matter how much money I make I never have enough."

Then identify the negative mental and emotional energy patterns involved by filling in the blanks like this: *No matter how much money I make I never have enough* because I believe _____ and this makes me feel _____. Look at how this pattern has played out throughout your life. When did you first start to think and feel this way? Finally, create an affirmation that reflects a new mental and emotional energy pattern for the situation. For instance: "I deserve to have what I need without worry or overwork. My works bring me rewards of abundance and joy." Create a mental picture of you living in the state your affirmation describes.

Don't Get Fooled by Energy Bars

Energy bars don't offer any more energy than eating other food with the same amount of calories. So says Lona Sandon, a spokesperson for the American Dietetic Association in the *Tufts Nutrition Newsletter*. And you may miss out on valuable nutrients like calcium and potassium if you choose an energy bar rather than fruits, vegetables, and dairy products. However, if the alternative is to skip eating altogether, they are better than nothing. Just be sure to check the label. You want to find ones that are 200 calories or less, low in fat, and with at least three grams of fiber. Take it with water so that you get the full fiber benefit. And to save money, instead of packing an energy bar, combine whole grain cereal, nuts, and dried fruit in a plastic bag and take it along with you for an energy snack.

ENERGY
BOOSTER

348

Go with the Flow

When someone comes toward you with strong energy, what do you do? Push back and defend yourself, which takes a tremendous amount of your energy? Attack their ideas? Collapse in helplessness? Take a tip from Aikido masters and go where the oncoming energy wants to go first. "Tell me more," you might say. "What else could I do differently or better?" The more you first receive his or her strong energy, the less energy you have to expend and the more he or she will then be willing to later hear your side.

This means learning not to be defensive, which can be challenging. Try doing it once, however, and we bet you'll feel so good about how effective and energy saving it is that soon it will be easy to do.

Manage Your Kids' Energy

In his book, *Transforming the Difficult Child*, Howard Glasser describes kids as energy junkies. They thrive on high energy—from TV, video games, and parents. And most kids get the most parental energy when they do something wrong. You go ballistic, and they get a free charge!

His solution: give high-energy positive reinforcement to behavior you want to see more of and low-energy discipline or punishment. When reprimanding, stay as energetically calm, neutral, and quiet as possible—"I told you, Madison, that you couldn't do that, so now you have to go to your room." Look for positive behavior to comment on in as rousing a way as possible. Soon your kids will do more of what you want and less of what you don't—and you won't have to exert so much effort!

Alternate Hot and Cold
in the Shower

This is a tried and true technique for waking up quickly. It boosts your metabolism and your circulation.

Take a Red-Light Break

When you're dog-tired and waiting at a traffic light, take a red-light break. Anyone can do it, but it's a special boon for parents of young children. Ask your kids to watch for the moment the light turns green. Meanwhile, shift the car into park, close your eyes, and relax into the seat. Exhale deeply and let a new breath fill you up. When you relax, you realize how much useless energy it takes to idly watch the cross traffic.

If you have many years of driving under your belt, you can usually predict when the light is about to change. But kids love to announce, "It's green, Mommy! Green!" They enjoy the grown-up responsibility; you enjoy the minibreak. And you both enjoy a rejuvenated parent.

ENERGY
BOOSTER

352

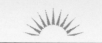

Decorate with Amber Hues

Color therapists say the color amber beats fatigue. Try amber votives or lamp shades, or orange candles, pillows, rugs. Or go wild with amber walls or carpet.

The Big Skinny

Can't tell if you're coming or going? A great way to regain which way you're headed is to explore the organ that gauges where you are in the world: your skin. Your skin is your body's largest organ—12 percent of your body weight and somewhere between twelve and twenty square feet if you laid it out on the carpet. It lets you know when you're near something or touching it, how you connect to the earth, what a hug feels like.

Notice where the surface of your skin meets the world. Perhaps you feel air cooling your face, the waistband of your pants, gravity pulling you toward the chair or floor. Your skin even lets light in—close your eyes and see the muted light permeating your eyelids. Your skin (along with your inner ear and sense of balance) tells you where you are in space—you can feel your hand on the book, your neck curling to read, where you are in a room or outdoors. Your skin senses the larger world, and it also separates you—the sensation beneath your epidermis is different than it feels on its surface. Knowing the difference between the inside and outside can harmonize busy times and help you to center yourself.

ENERGY
BOOSTER

354

Change the Words on Your Computer

Eye stress makes us feel tired, even when the rest of the body is humming along. And computer staring (working, surfing, playing games) can tax the vision. A simple way to reduce eye strain is to change the type size on your computer screen. With smaller type your eyes may scrunch, you may lean forward to see, and you may have too much information to absorb on a page. With too-large type, you may not read as quickly (we mostly read by paragraphs and sentences, not word by word) and you may have to spend time scrolling to new pages.

You can use computer glasses to ease your eyes, but play with your computer programs before an optometrist visit. In software that runs graphics, word or data processing, you can increase the font size itself—just make sure the type looks right on a printed copy. Or you can adjust the monitor view by changing the Zoom command in the View menu, or the Zoom percentage on the toolbar (from a tiny 10 percent to a huge 500 percent of the printed copy). On Internet programs, change the type size for most Web sites in the View menu/Text Size control. If you're familiar with your computer's operating systems (or know someone who can help), you can make other monitor updates: With an LCD (flat panel) monitor, turn on ClearType which makes the fonts look smoother. With a CRT (regular monitor), increase video refresh frequency to greater than the 60 Hz default setting; video refresh is how frequently the screen gets redrawn, and the 60 Hz default can flicker in some people's peripheral vision.

Get Cozy

The feeling of coziness can bring renewal to fast-paced days. Think of "cozy" as accepting your natural body rhythms. Set aside some private and uninterrupted time—ten minutes will work, thirty is even better. Get a cozy thing you like to do—a favorite book, a new catalog, music, people watching. Find a place—the bathtub, a blanket on a couch, a favorite coffee shop. Settle in, breathe, relax your muscles.

Your job is simple: Be your own cozy buddy and follow your natural inclination. Do you read for a while then day-dream? Do you like to switch songs on CDs or listen to the whole album? Do candles, or doodling, or watching out your window make you feel at home with your pace? Follow how your body wants to be cozy today. Tomorrow your coziness may be different. Snuggle into yourself.

Soften Your Brain

Your brain works hard; your skull holds on to your working brain; your body and shoulders support your working skull. Do you need to work hard to think well? What if even your brain relaxed? The consistency of your brain is actually quite soft, like a raw egg. During meditation, the brain waves change to alpha and theta—and perhaps the consistency of the brain softens. Imagining a softer brain gives a sense of release, lets your shoulders relax, and changes your pattern of thinking.

Take a moment to notice your head and brain. Feel the muscles of the face and skull. Imagine the brain under that round dome, and let it relax. Visualize a space between the skull and brain. Or feel as if the brain has the consistency of soft butter. Or hear your brain gently humming. Or say, "My soft brain relaxes." If touching helps, place one hand on the forehead and one on the base of the skull. A moment of brain relaxation—a break after all its hard work.

Play a Game

What is it about puzzles and games that relaxes and stimulates us? Studies show that exercising your brain staves off Alzheimer's disease, helps promote spatial orientation, and in the case of bridge or other card games, creates community connections. When your brain works better, your thinking power takes you farther on less mental gas.

Puzzles and games—crosswords, jigsaws, word games—help you take a break from the day-to-day grind. You become immersed in meeting a challenge. You get a sense of accomplishment—perhaps creativity. And with some card games, you create order out of chaos. Something you can't always do at home.

Encourage your own mental challenges, and let your brain continue to grow.

Write It Off

Writing changes your perspective and helps you solve problems. All it requires is ten minutes (use a clock or timer to stay focused), a paper, and pen. The movement of your hand on paper gives words a flow. On a computer, people tend to edit as they write. With paper and pen, you can get more juice because you can't change what you've said, you just keep going. If you blank out when you see a sheet of white paper, don't worry about your eighth grade English teacher. This is just for you. Write the story that's on your mind. Or write phrases that describe important parts of the story—who, where, what, when, feelings.

Writing changes your perspective when you discover something new. One way is to answer some questions as you write: What have I done in this situation? What would I still like to do? What do I know? What don't I know? Your pen might unleash some wisdom you hadn't expected, and with it some energy.

Stay Away from
the Computer at Night

If you love playing on the computer before bedtime, you may be keeping yourself up at night. A Japanese study researched why computer-game players have later bedtimes and shorter sleep hours. They discovered that gamers produced less of the hormone melatonin, which is linked to sleep. Researchers surmise that gazing at a brightly lit display while performing an exciting task affects the human biological clock. Might be true of late-night TV watching as well. Give yourself some darker, calmer wind-down time before hitting the hay.

Just the Way You Are

Some of us use our energy and intelligence on how we appear—worrying over bad hair, body weight, the most striking clothes. A study showed that people who spent lots of time adjusting their hair, clothing, or appearance had less intelligence for other tasks. Worries and frets can get in the way of what's really important. And we like to look good. How to resolve that inner dialogue about how we appear?

A simple way is to answer the worries—out loud. For example, Diane fretted about a bad hair day. To answer her qualms over something that wouldn't change that day, she'd say, "This is how my hair looks today, Diane, and it is just fine." Say your phrase aloud in a loving and firm voice, and mention your name. You might say it to yourself into a mirror. And you really are just fine.

L-Tyrosine and Amino Acids

Sometimes a lack of attention can make daily lives more stressful and tiresome. Important events or information might get lost in the mind. Perhaps it's information overload, tiredness, ADD, or another peculiarity in how brains work. Author Daniel Amen (*www.brainplace.com*) explores the tendencies of brains and methods to handle them, from exercise to medicine to nutrition. One suggestion for ADD-type symptoms is the amino acid L-tyrosine.

Amino acids, building blocks for protein, are essential for the body's digestion, cell repair, overall metabolism, and the development of the brain. The amino acid L-tyrosine helps create the neurotransmitter dopamine—an essential element of thinking and concentration in the prefrontal cortex of the brain. Dr. Amen prescribes 500–1500 milligrams of L-tyrosine two to three times per day for adults, on an empty stomach. Check with your doctor and the Brainplace Web site for more information on how to determine your brain type and if L-tyrosine is right for you. You may discover that another amino acid or brain supplement strategy helps better clear your thinking.

Smudging Sage

People have been burning dried plants for millennia as a way to release fragrant energy. The ritual of smudging—the name comes from Native American culture—can create feelings of healing and balancing, and some say the smoke dissipates unneeded or old energies.

Many dried plants can be smudged—such as sage, cedar, red willow bark, juniper, lavender, and sweet grass. Sage *Artemisia*—white sage or garden sage (not the cooking herb *Salvia*)—has become popular for smudging, for clearing out old energy and moving on to the new. You can buy tied bundles of the dried herb at health food stores, some bookstores, and on the Web. There are many old and new rites for smudging, and you can invent your own. One simple way is to light the sage until it starts to smoke, then take it near the corners of the rooms you want to refresh.

Or you can sage yourself or a friend. Bring the lit sage up from your feet to your scalp (both front and back). You might make small circles at spots that feel tense, or if you are familiar with the points of energy on the body, chakras, you can pause or circle there. At the end, you can "zip yourself up" moving the lit sage in a line from near your feet to just at the top of your head. To put the sage out, you can press the embers on a seashell, earthen pottery, or a jar of sand.

Exhale Deeply

We tend to think of taking a deep breath as the route to revitalization, but it's important to take a deep exhale first—out with the old to make room for the new.

Give it a try right now—breathe out a little longer than normally. Now a little longer, and longer still. There's a lot of stagnant air hiding in the bronchioles of your lungs. In a normal exhale, we get rid of only about 15 percent of the air in our lungs. Getting it out means there's more room for vitalizing oxygen to get in.

A natural reaction to stress is to inhale or breathe shallowly. A deep exhale (perhaps even with a little hiss at the end forcing air from every cranny) makes the next inhale naturally deep and relaxed. Instantly you will be more alert.

Review the Day

The day can become so busy with errands, meetings, conversations, and thoughts, we feel unfinished in the evening. Like a sentence that needs a period. Sleep can tie up some loose ends. But you can "unburden" sleep by reviewing the day before bed.

Settle into your bed or a chair, and rest into your body. Then consider your day, starting from the morning to evening, or in reverse. Include areas of concern, things unfinished or accomplished, what gave you joy, what made you grateful.

The day's review is like looking at yourself on your life's map. Where did you travel today? Where might you want to go tomorrow? Appreciate the journey.

BIBLIOGRAPHY

Daniel Amen. *Healing the Hardware of the Soul*. New York: Simon and Schuster, 2003.

Martha Beck. "Ready . . . Aim . . . Oh Well . . ." *O*, July 2003.

Herbert Benson and Miriam Z. Klipper. *The Relaxation Response*. New York: Avon, 2000.

Emily Bergeron. "Cracking the Energy Bar Code." *Tufts Daily*, April 2004.

www.bettersleep.org.

Julia Cameron. *The Artist's Way*. New York: Tarcher/Penguin, 2002.

Don Campbell. *The Mozart Effect: Tapping the Power of Music to Heal the Body, Strengthen the Mind, and Unlock the Creative Spirit*. New York: Quill, 2001.

Rick Carson. *Taming Your Gremlin*. New York: Quill, 2003.

Bern S. Cherewatenko and Paul Perry. *The Stress Cure*. New York: HarperResource, 2003.

Marla Cilley. *Sink Reflections*. New York: Bantam Books, 2002.

Brenda Davies. *Chakra Power Beads*. Berkeley, CA: Ulysses Press, 2001.

www.dremilykane.com (Dr. Emily Kane's naturopathic articles).

www.drweil.com (Dr. Andrew Weil, alternative medicine).

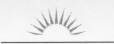

Donna Eden. *Energy Medicine*. New York: Tarcher/Penguin, 1999.

Sharon Goldman Edry. "Stress? Get Away." *Health*, April 2003.

"Energy Makeovers." *O*, July 2003.

Adele Faber and Elaine Mazlish. *How to Talk So Kids Will Listen and Listen So Kids Will Talk*. New York: Quill, 2004.

Tapas Fleming. *You Can Heal Now*. Redondo Beach, CA: TAT International, 1999.

www.flylady.com (organizing your home).

Susan Gilmore. "How to Calm the Traffic Waves." *The Seattle Times*, October 6, 2002.

Rosemary Gladstar. *Family Herbal*. North Adams, MA: Storey Books, 2001.

Jim Gordon. *Become an Energy Addict*. Atlanta, GA: Longstreet Press, 2003.

Edward Hallowell. *Worry*. New York: Ballantine, 1998.

Jesse Lynn Hanley and Nancy Deville. *Tired of Being Tired*. New York: G. P. Putnam and Sons, 2001.

Naura Hayden. *Everything You've Always Wanted to Know about Energy But Were Too Weak to Ask*. New York: Bibli O-Phile Publishing Company, 1993.

Dana Hudepohl. "Are You Tired All the Time?" *Cosmopolitan*, June 2002.

www.iSleepless.Com (sleep disorders).

Gregg D. Jacobs. *Say Good Night to Insomnia*. New York: Henry Holt and Company, 1999.

Jon Kabot-Zinn. *Full Catastrophe Living*. New York: Delta, 1990.

Amy Rapaport Karlson. "62 Ways to Feel Great Naturally." *Natural Health*, May/June 2003.

Byron Katie. *Loving What Is: Four Questions That Can Change Your Life*. New York: Crown Publishing Group, 2002.

Donald Kaufman and Taffy Dahl. *Color: Natural Palettes for Painted Rooms*. New York: Crown Publishing Group, 1992.

Chris Kilham. "Siberia's Golden Herbs." *Prevention*, February 2003.

Tae Yun Kim. *The First Element*. Milpitas, CA: Northstar, 1999.

Janet Kinosian. *The Well-Rested Woman*. York Beach, ME: Red Wheel/Weiser, 2002.

Mira Kirshenbaum. *The Emotional Energy Factor*. New York: Delacorte, 2003.

Jack Kornfield. *After the Ecstasy, the Laundry*. New York: Bantam Books, 2001.

Sue Kovach. *Healing Herbs to Keep You Out of the Doctor's Office*. Boca Raton, FL: American Media Mini Mags, 2002.

Barbara and Kevin Kunz. *My Reflexologist Says Feet Don't Lie*. Albuquerque, NM: Reflexology Research Project, 2001.

Kathryn Perrotti Leavitt. "Outwit 7 Hidden Energy Sappers." *Natural Health*, May/June 2003.

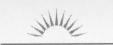

Sue Lilly and Simon Lilly. *Crystal Healing*. London: Lorenz Books, 2002.

Denise Linn. *Sacred Space*. New York: Ballantine Books, 1995.

Jim Loehr and Tony Schwartz. *The Power of Full Engagement*. New York: Free Press, 2003.

Elisa Lottor. and Nancy P. Bruning. *Female and Forgetful*. New York: Warner Books, 2002.

Craig Mardus. *How to Make Worry Work for You*. New York: Warner Books, 1995.

www.mcphee.com (Archie McPhee's toys and amusements).

Susan McQuillan. "Your Ultimate Energy Diet." *Fitness*, June 2002.

Ragini Elizabeth Michaels. *Facticity*. Seattle, WA: Facticity Trainings, Inc., 1991.

Cullen Murphy. "Hello, Darkness: Dealing with Yet Another Deficit." *Atlantic Monthly*, March 1996.

www.napo.net (National Association of Professional Organizers).

www.nia-nia.com (Neuromuscular Integrative Action: freestyle meditative dance).

www.officeplayground.com (desk gizmos and toys).

Suzannah Oliver. *101 Ways to Stress-Free Living*. London: Friedman/Fairfax, 2003.

Judith Orloff. *Positive Energy*. New York: Harmony, 2004.

Suze Orman. *Courage to Be Rich*. New York: Penguin Group, 2001.

Katherine Paterson. *The Bridge to Terabithia*. New York: HarperCollins Children's Book Group, 1987.

Karen Patterson. "Research Shows Green Views can Alleviate Stress, Boost Attention." *The Dallas Morning News*, April 9, 2004.

www.prairiehome.publicradio.org (Garrison Keillor, *A Prairie Home Companion*).

www.prevention.com.

www.purewhitenoise.com (white noise CDs and machines).

Lorin Roche. *Meditation Made Easy*. New York: Harper San Francisco, 1998.

Nic Rowley, et al. *Energize Your Life*. New York: One Spirit, 2001.

www.sleepmachines.com (white noise CDs and machines).

Pamela Smith. *The Energy Edge*. New York: HarperResource, 1999.

Annette Spence. "Iron Out Your Intake." *Delicious Living*, May 2002.

Robert E. Thayer. *Calm Energy*. Oxford, England: Oxford University Press, 2001.

www.washingtonpost.com/wp-dyn/liveonline/style/tellmeaboutit (Carolyn Hax chat and advice).

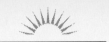

Debra Waterhouse. *Outsmarting Female Fatigue*. New York: Hyperion, 2001.

Andrew Weil. *Eight Weeks to Optimum Health*. New York: Ballantine Books, 1998.

E. B.White. *Charlotte's Web*. New York: Harper Trophy, 1974.

Ruth White. *Using Your Chakras*. York Beach, ME: Samuel Weiser, 1998.

Laura Whitworth, Henry Kimsey-House, and Phil Sandahl. *Co-Active Coaching*. Palo Alto, CA: Consulting Psychologists Press, 1998.

ABOUT THE AUTHORS

Susannah Seton is the author of the Simple Pleasures series, including *Simple Pleasures*, *Simple Pleasures of the Garden*, *Simple Pleasures of Home*, *Simple Pleasures for the Holidays*, *365 Simple Pleasures*, *Simple Pleasures of the Kitchen*, and *Simple Pleasures of Friendship*. She lives in the San Francisco Bay Area.

Sondra Kornblatt is a writer, life coach, and originator of Creative Insomnia. She has published articles on wellness, spirituality, and parenting in magazines and Web sites, including *ParentMap* and *Seattle's Child*. Previously she was publisher at Group Health Publishing and worked on health information projects at Microsoft. She teaches Creative Insomnia, a technique she developed for finding inner renewal at night—even while awake. As a life coach she helps clients with their dreams, career, and wellness for happier days and nights. She can be reached at *www.CreativeInsomnia.com*.

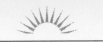

To Our Readers

Conari Press, an imprint of Red Wheel/Weiser, publishes books on topics ranging from spirituality, personal growth, and relationships to women's issues, parenting, and social issues. Our mission is to publish quality books that will make a difference in people's lives—how we feel about ourselves and how we relate to one another. We value integrity, compassion, and receptivity, both in the books we publish and in the way we do business.

Our readers are our most important resource, and we value your input, suggestions, and ideas about what you would like to see published. Please feel free to contact us, to request our latest book catalog, or to be added to our mailing list.

Conari Press
An imprint of Red Wheel/Weiser, LLC
P.O. Box 612
York Beach, ME 03910-0612
www.conari.com